A LOVE FOR LIFE

Jane & Glenn McGrath

A LOVE
FOR LIFE

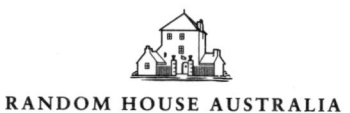

RANDOM HOUSE AUSTRALIA

Random House Australia Pty Ltd
20 Alfred Street, Milsons Point, NSW 2061
http://www.randomhouse.com.au

Sydney   New York   Toronto
London   Auckland   Johannesburg

First published by Random House Australia 2000
Copyright © Jane and Glenn McGrath 2000

All rights reserved. No part of this publication may be reproduced, stored in a retrieval system, or transmitted in any form or by any means, electronic, mechanical, photocopying, recording or otherwise, without the prior written permission of the publisher.

National Library of Australia
Cataloguing-in-Publication Entry

McGrath, Jane and Glenn.
A Love for Life.

ISBN 0 09184 153 4

1. McGrath, Jane. 2. McGrath, Glenn. 3. Breast – Cancer – Patients – Australia – Biography.
4. Mastectomy – Patients – Australia – Biography. 5. Cricket players – Australia – Biography.
I. McGrath, Glenn. II. title.
362.196994490092

Internal design by Gayna Murphy
Typeset in Bell MT 13.5/16 and Bell Gothic 12.5/16 by Midland Typesetters, Maryborough, Victoria
Printed and bound by Griffin Press, Netley, South Australia

10 9 8 7 6 5 4 3 2

For our darling son James,
proof that dreams can come true—never give up.

CONTENTS

Foreword ix

Part 1 Early Days 1
In the Beginning 3
Love Blossoms 33
Love Hurts 52

Part 2 Our New Life 59
A Fearful Discovery 61
A Turning Point 90
Blackest Days 100
The Fight Goes On 121

Part 3 Happy Ever After 145
On Top of the World 147
Wedding Bells 163
A Dream Come True 169
Epilogue 176

Acknowledgements 178
What Should I Look Out For? 179
Contacts and Resources 180

FOREWORD

Having arrived in Sydney from the UK in 1994 myself, I knew exactly how hard it was to leave your family, friends and career behind and move to the other side of the world to be with someone you hardly knew, never mind that that person wouldn't be in the same country as you most of the time. When Jane arrived in Australia, I was a veteran, so I took her under my wing.

It was really exciting to be with someone who could give me an update on all the English soaps—*Eastenders, Brookside* and *Coronation Street!* We would talk for hours about the antics of Curly Watts, what Tiff and Grant were doing and who was our favourite chef on *Ready Steady Cook*—all very important topics!

Life had always seemed a struggle when Michael left for a tour but after Jane arrived, it became much easier.

I will never forget the day Jane came into my hotel room during the 1997 Ashes tour. She told me she'd found a lump in her breast. I made light of it, but told her to go and get it checked out, to put her mind at rest. In the end, she decided she would wait until she returned to Oz the following week.

Michael and I stayed on in England for a two-week holiday at the end of the Ashes tour but I called Jane as soon as we returned to Sydney. She told me the devastating news that the lump she had found was in fact much more than just a lump; she had breast cancer and needed a mastectomy in order to save her life.

My head was spinning at such terrible news. I felt nauseous, and just wanted to put the phone down, go to her, put my arms around her and tell her everything was going to be alright. My best friend, the person I had only known for such a short time yet felt was my sister, the person I had already spent so many days with, laughing, joking, telling all my secrets to—it had to be a cruel mistake. She was too young to have cancer.

I have never really been a religious person, but I found myself saying a prayer every night, asking for an angel to look after my very special friend.

I had always thought I was a strong person, but I now know what true strength is. I watched Jane go through her operation, chemotherapy and radiotherapy, and never once did I hear her ask 'Why me?'

The average person in the street would never have guessed that the beautiful blue-eyed blonde wearing the tight-fitting tops and jeans was fighting one of life's toughest battles.

I believe things happen for a reason, and I had thought Jane had come into my life to be the friend I thought I would never have in Australia. I now know that Jane came into my life to show me what real life is all about, what real problems are, how very precious life is and how so many of us take it for granted. She has shown me what a positive attitude is, what real inner strength is, and I feel truly blessed having her in my life.

One of my happiest days was when I was Matron of

FOREWORD

Honour at Glenn and Jane's wedding. It meant so much to me to see her looking so beautiful and healthy and finally marrying the man I knew she loved more than anyone in this world, the man who had been her reason to fight the terrible disease that had invaded her body.

I think the only other time I have cried so much (apart from my own wedding day and the birth of our daughter Olivia) was the day she told me she was pregnant. That was the icing on the cake!

I am proud to say that Jane is Olivia's godmother. Who better to guide our precious little girl through life than Jane?

Tracy Bevan

Part One

EARLY DAYS

IN THE BEGINNING

When I was diagnosed with breast cancer, at thirty-one years of age, my life changed forever.

Losing a breast at any age seemed to me to be a fate worse than death, something I could hardly bear to even imagine. In the past, when I'd heard people say that, for one reason or another, their lives had been 'turned upside down' or that their 'world had come crashing down around them', I'd thought I was able to put myself in their position and imagine how they must have felt. It wasn't until I was diagnosed with breast cancer on Wednesday, 10 September 1997 that I truly realised what it felt like to have your life turned upside down and your entire world come crashing down, leaving you feeling completely powerless to do anything to stop it. Not only was it an attack on my life, but also on my womanhood; my femininity.

But let me go back to the beginning. I was born on 4 May 1966, in Staffordshire, a fairly green county in the Midlands of England. I did most of my growing up in what was then a small town called Brownhills, about a 10-minute drive from the countryside in one direction but a 30-minute drive from the industrial areas of Birmingham and Walsall in the opposite direction. Dad's parents and his sister lived in Walsall and we'd go and visit them most weekends. Mum's parents, Sidney and Emily Kendrick, lived in Brownhills for most of their lives. My grandad was an orphan, and from the age of fifteen, he worked with my great-grandfather down the coal mine. My great-grandfather took pity on him and brought Grandad home to live with him and his family. That was when he first met my nan—she was thirteen then. It wasn't love at first sight—in fact Nan hated him—but slowly love blossomed. In later life, Grandad was a bricklayer. He loved horse racing, and his favourite pastime was studying the form guide and having a bet on the gee gees, as he called them. Whenever he went out, be it for dinner or just to fetch the newspaper, he'd never be without a shirt with a collar and his trilby. Sadly, this lovely man died in July 1985. My memories of him are all great ones. Nan used to run the greengrocers in Brownhills' High Street—every-one knew Emily Kendrick.

Mum and Dad met when they worked together at the Gas Board and married soon after. Mum was twenty-one. Dad then went into partnership with Nan and they ran the shop together. A few years later, Nan bought a sweet shop, which my younger brother Jonathan and I thought was just fantastic! It had jars and jars of sweets covering the shelves behind the counter, and every chocolate bar ever made. Then there were all the halfpenny and penny sweets and lucky bags on the counter in front. I thought it was simply heaven. I think that must be where I acquired my very sweet tooth!

Growing up in Brownhills I played the usual girly games with my friends, like squishing up rose petals in water to make our own very special perfume, making up dance routines and pretending we were a '70s dance troupe on *Top of the Pops*, and—my personal favourite—dressing up and parading up and down the road in our mums' shoes pretending we were about twenty-five years old and thinking we looked pretty good! Another one of my favourite pastimes, which may seem a little strange, involved an old toothbrush and a bowl of water. On a sunny day, I would love nothing more than sitting in the back garden with toothbrush in hand scrubbing the garden paving slabs clean. I derived immense satisfaction from seeing them look shiny and new by the end of the afternoon.

Mum and Dad divorced, amicably, when I was eleven, and although Jon and I lived with Mum, we only lived about five minutes away from Dad. We stayed with him twice a week, so it wasn't too bad, for us at least. I remember their divorce quite clearly, and feel I coped with it well, though it did make me grow up quickly. I remember feeling terribly sorry for Dad, as I felt he now had no one to look after him, so I would take it upon myself to clean his house after school and make him packet trifles to keep his strength up.

Mum and Dad being divorced did make me think that I would never get married. I'd seen my parents' marriage break up and that, coupled with the fact that I felt I would never meet anyone I loved or trusted enough to even contemplate spending the rest of my life with, let alone have them feel the same way about me, left me believing I would always be single. It wasn't something I ever lost any sleep over—it was just the way I felt. I had friends who kept scrapbooks full of clippings and ideas for their wedding day. When the time came, they would know exactly what they wanted. It was something I never gave a moment's thought to.

I've always been a very healthy person, although not what you could call sporty. I was usually one of the last to be chosen when a school team was being selected for hockey or netball. I was quite small in those days and not at all athletic. As for cricket, I don't recall us even having a school cricket team. In fact, I couldn't even tell you what sports the boys played—I wasn't interested. However, I did take an interest in football (soccer, as it's known as down under). My brother was, and still is, an ardent Aston Villa supporter and I used to follow Liverpool, partly because my best friend at the time did and partly because they had quite a few handsome players! I knew absolutely nothing about cricket back then and didn't care. I always pictured it as a rather boring sport watched mainly by old people. As Tracy Bevan once said, she thought a cricket match was where old people went to die. I never dreamed that one day it would be such a big part of my life.

Now if there was a school quiz, I was your girl. My strengths most definitely lay inside the classroom rather than outside on the sports field. At junior (primary) school, I absolutely loved reading, and was a real bookworm. I always wanted to be Enid Blyton when I grew up.

From what I can gather, Australian children appear to spend far more time outside and playing sport than I did, which I think is great. Australians seem to be players of sport rather than observers, unlike the English. I frequently have this argument with Mark Waugh, who delights in letting me know how bad he thinks the English are at sport—all sport. I can't wait for the day when England beat Australia at something. (Please let it be soon and not cricket.) England is quite good at sports like darts, dominoes and snooker—anything you can play at the pub. There seems to be a far greater variety of sports and outdoor pursuits in Australia than in England, and of course the weather is a hundred times better than in England. I think the Australian

IN THE BEGINNING

way of life is simply a much healthier lifestyle altogether.

As a teenager, I was more interested in the latest fashions and music than sport. It was around that time when New Romantic bands like Duran Duran, Human League and Depeche Mode were really popular. It was all black eyeliner, pedal pushers, frilly shirts and long scarves with lots of lurex and tassels on the end that you'd swirl around as you danced at the local disco—and that was just the blokes! The girls were all in ra-ra skirts that were short on one side and long on the other with a double belt slung somewhere across the body. When I think back to some of the clothes I used to wear, I can't believe Mum ever let me out of the house. She used to call my skirts pelmets, they were so short. One Friday night, my friend Julie and I managed to blag our way into a nightclub called The Rum Runner in Birmingham, which was where Duran Duran hung out. We were about sixteen, and we thought we looked pretty good. I remember seeing John Taylor (the bass player with Duran Duran) in there and I nearly went to pieces, until I got closer. He was wearing leather trousers that just hung off him, and he was so thin and spotty—I was crushed.

I have always been active and loved being outside in the fresh air, but to me keeping fit meant aerobics classes and gym sessions. I was as fit as a fiddle up until the age of fifteen, when I caught glandular fever right in the middle of my exam preparations. The doctors originally thought I might have meningitis, so to be diagnosed with glandular fever was quite a relief. It stuffed up my career plans, though, as I had hoped to go to university to study languages—French and German. I ended up being away from school for several months, so I had to come up with a career plan B instead. Rather than re-sit the year of schooling I missed out on, I decided to forego uni and go to technical college, where

I discovered I could do a similar course but leave with a slightly lesser qualification. When I left college, I quickly found out that few companies were prepared to employ an 18-year-old inexperienced bilingual secretary. In order to gain some experience and earn a bit of money at the same time, I started doing secretarial temping in Birmingham.

I enjoyed temping because each assignment was different— different locations, different work and meeting new people all the time, which really suited me as I have a tendency to get bored quite quickly. It was during one of my temping assignments that I heard the other girls in the office talking about a large local holiday company that was looking to take on overseas representatives to work in European resorts. I was ready for a change of scenery, and as the company's headquarters were only five minutes away from where I was working, I decided to apply for the position.

After a couple of interviews I was lucky enough to get the job. I was put on a training course with five other girls for a couple of weeks and then we were given our allocated resorts. I had been given the southern Spanish resort of Mojacar, as had a couple of the other girls on my training course. (How I ended up getting the Spanish assignment when my languages were French and German I'll never know.) I was twenty years old at the time and nursing a broken heart having just split up with my first boyfriend— we had been together for almost four years. It was the perfect opportunity for me to get away and do something new. When I was fourteen, I'd been lucky enough to go on a school skiing trip to the Dolomites in Italy, so I'd been away from home before, but this was the first time I'd been away from home and travelled to a new country without really knowing a soul. I was a little nervous but very excited.

I remember first arriving at the tiny Almeria airport in

IN THE BEGINNING

April. The first thing that hit me was the heat. As I walked off the plane on to the tarmac with the other girls from my course, it felt as though someone was holding a hairdryer in my face, a sensation I'd never experienced before! The other resort reps were there to meet us, and they directed us to our transport. The coach journey to the resort took about an hour, along very narrow mountain roads with sheer drops of hundreds of feet. The scenery was breathtaking. As we approached Mojacar, it looked just as it did in the holiday brochures—it was a fairly small village, with clusters of little white houses scattered over a hillside. The houses were covered in fuchsia-coloured bougainvillea and had orange and lemon trees in their little gardens—it was the first time I had seen such fruits actually growing on a tree, instead of in a little net bag in the supermarket.

In comparison to other Spanish resorts, Mojacar was small and quiet. There were a couple of nightclubs and seafood restaurants and some good beach bars, but the resort was mainly geared towards couples and families, not the 18–30 mob. This didn't stop the waiters, though. It was amazing to watch them surveying the new arrivals every week, searching out their prey and then swinging into action come nightfall. The poor little English girls didn't stand a chance against these Spanish romeos—mind you, I didn't hear many complaining. I watched it all from a distance, flabbergasted at how the same old corny lines managed to work week after week!

Part of my job was guiding excursions to local places of interest such as the nearby fishing port and traditional Spanish market town which had lots of little tapas bars centred mainly around the village square, where the older local men would sit in the cool shade and play chess or cards. I found I really enjoyed getting on the microphone at the front of the bus and filling the tourists in on local landmarks and customs. One of my favourite trips was to the beautiful old city of Granada with the magnificent Alhambra palace. It was such a popular excursion, the reps would queue up to guide it despite the fact that it was at least a four-hour journey to Granada from Mojacar and the coaches left at the crack of dawn. The architecture and gardens in the palace were absolutely amazing.

Those were the good sides to the job. When I took those away, I found I wasn't really enjoying my work very much at all. Apart from the intense heat from the Mediterranean sun which, English rose that I am, I struggled with daily, I felt I was just someone the holidaymakers came and moaned to. They'd rarely come up to tell you what a fantastic holiday they were having or just have a chat. It wasn't my idea of fun. After five months in Mojacar I decided it was time to find something new.

Having decided to leave Mojacar, I was interested when one of the other reps there said to me that she'd heard that a new London-based airline called Virgin Atlantic was recruiting flight attendants and that maybe I should give it a go. It was a job I'd never given a single thought to until that moment but it sounded fantastic. She had a contact at Virgin and gave me a name and telephone number to call and so, with nothing to lose, I gave them a ring. Virgin said they'd send me an application form so I handed in my notice, flew back home to England and submitted my application. It seemed to be an eternity before I heard anything back. It was only a week or so, but by now I wanted the job so badly I was running to the letterbox to get the post every morning. I pictured myself having coffee with my friends, discussing what we'd do that weekend, and me telling them that sorry, I wouldn't be able to see them that weekend as I was flying to

IN THE BEGINNING

New York and then Los Angeles the week after! I wondered if I'd ever be lucky enough to find myself in that position. I was absolutely thrilled when I finally received a letter from Virgin stating that I'd been selected to attend for an interview.

Interviews are nerve-racking at the best of times, but I felt this one was even more so. Apart from wanting to say the right things, I knew that Virgin's grooming standards were very high, and I desperately wanted to look my best. When I'd been travelling, I'd noticed that lots of flight attendants were wearing their hair in a French plait, so I thought I'd at least try to look the part and do the same. One visit to the hairdresser later I was on my way to where the interview was to take place—a hotel near Gatwick airport, about a three-hour journey south from Mum's, so my good friend (who's also called Jane) travelled with me for company and some moral support.

When it was time for my interview and my name was called, I turned to Jane, seeking some reassurance, and asked her how I looked. 'Like a tennis ball,' she replied, giggling. My plait was too tight! It was not quite the response I'd been looking for. I wanted to cry. However, despite my resemblance to said tennis ball, I got the job, and my career in the skies took off on 10 July 1989, when I began a five-week intensive training course. Virgin are extremely hot on aircraft flight safety and first aid, and their training course reflected this. Even now, whenever I fly I find myself looking around to see if the galley's secure and everything's been locked and stowed correctly in the cabin.

We had to do firefighting at a mock-up aircraft at Gatwick airport. This involved entering a smoke-filled chamber wearing breathing apparatus, finding the fire and extinguishing it. We also had to carry out a ditching drill in the Training

Centre swimming pool. This involved clambering in and out of life rafts, getting extremely wet in the process.

However, of all the demands made of a flight attendant during training, my absolute least favourite was having to jump down the door evacuation slide. Most of the others in my group looked upon it as a ride at Wonderland, but I just couldn't see it that way. It wasn't the height of the drop or length of the slide that was the problem. It was the fact that you couldn't just sit down on it and slide down. Oh no, because it was a mock emergency evacuation, you had to almost run and jump onto the slide, and there was nothing to hold on to. One by one, the rest of my training course jumped down it. I just kept edging to the back of the queue. Eventually I was the only one left, but I still couldn't bring myself to jump—my feet were glued! Of course by now everyone else was at the bottom of the slide, watching my every move and urging me to jump, shouting to me that it was great fun. I didn't believe them. The instructor took me to one side, away from the door and the sheer drop, and explained, kindly but firmly, that if I didn't jump, I would fail the course. The pressure to jump had suddenly increased a hundredfold, but I was still having problems with the concept. In the end, the instructor walked me down to the back door (where the incline of the slide is steeper, by the way), said he'd count to three and I would either have to jump or go home. He got to two and I went, screaming all the way down the slide.

At the end of the course, there was a Safety and Emergency Procedures (SEP) examination, for which the pass mark was 88 per cent. There was a lot of studying during that five weeks, but I'm happy to say I passed and soon I had started my new career as a flight attendant. It was all really exciting and I absolutely loved flying. There was so much variety. Every flight was different—different destination,

IN THE BEGINNING

different crew, different passengers. For someone who gets bored as easily as I do, life as a flight attendant was just perfect. No two days were ever the same. Virgin was a relatively new and quite small airline, and the majority of the crew were young and really enthusiastic. When I was with them, they flew mainly to the US—New York, Miami, LA, Boston, Orlando, San Francisco, Washington—but also to Moscow, Tokyo and Hong Kong.

On a jumbo jet, you'd have (on average) fifteen cabin crew plus two or three flight deck crew. Each time you flew (which was usually about five times a month), you'd fly with different crew, which meant you were working with and meeting new people all the time, which I loved. I made some great friends flying, several of whom are still good friends now. Two of my close 'Virgin' friends flew out to Sydney for our wedding. In fact one of them, Lorraine, was a bridesmaid and the other, Anna, did a reading for us. It was wonderful to have them there.

Because I flew mainly out of Heathrow, I decided to move down to London, and I ended up living there for five years. During that time, I lived in a few different areas of London—Chiswick, Greenwich, Marble Arch and Highbury, the home of the Arsenal football team, otherwise known as 'the Gunners'. It was a handy place to live for me, because the tube station at Highbury was on the Piccadilly line, which took me straight to Heathrow. The downside was that the Arsenal team plays in a red strip and my Virgin uniform was also red. Getting home from a flight on a Saturday afternoon (match day) was an absolute nightmare, not to mention ever so slightly embarrassing. I used to feel like the team mascot, dressed in red from head to toe, completely worn out—I'd been up all night walking across the Atlantic—and having to drag my suitcase through the throngs of excited and, on occasion, somewhat inebriated Arsenal supporters all going in the opposite direction to me.

Flying gave me some great opportunities to see the world. Some of the longer trips we did meant we were away for several days—it was just like being on a mini holiday. When I first started with Virgin, there were five-night Orlando trips, so we got to go to Disney World and Sea World. On one occasion, I was lucky enough to be there when a space shuttle was scheduled to take off. My friend and I hired a car and drove off to Cape Canaveral to get a closer look. Without doubt, though, my most frequently visited destination was the Big Apple, and even though I must have seen the Manhattan skyline countless times, it always brought a smile to my face.

One of the sights I feel most privileged to have seen is the aurora borealis, otherwise known as the Northern Lights. It's a natural phenomenon best viewed a fair way north—the closer to Greenland and the Arctic Circle the better. Being eight kilometres up in the air means you get a pretty clear unpolluted view, too! Generally, the 'lights' are white, but on occasion they can be different colours. One night we were returning to London from New York in the very early hours of the morning. I was working on the Upper Deck, and all of my passengers were sleeping soundly. My Supervisor came out of the Flight Deck laughing that the Captain had asked if she wanted to see the Northern Lights as they were particularly good that night, the best he'd ever seen. It was evident from her reaction that she couldn't have cared less about seeing them, but I was so excited about this rare opportunity that I immediately went rushing into the Flight Deck to see what all the fuss was about. I was so enthusiastic, the Captain thought I'd been sent in as a joke. I raced back to the galley, returning quickly with tea and cookies, and stayed in there for about half an hour witnessing the most fantastic natural laser show ever while the Captain explained to me what it was all about.

During my seven years with Virgin, one of my favourite experiences was when I and three of my friends decided to visit Australia for a six-week holiday backpacking up the east coast, from Sydney to Cairns. I'd never been backpacking before and, to be honest, I didn't know if I really fancied it, but it sounded like a great adventure so I put my name down.

We arrived in Sydney in March 1994, and ended up staying at a hostel in Kings Cross, which I now know isn't the most salubrious part of town. However we didn't know this at the time. It was colourful, to say the least. I love watching bands play live and couldn't believe it when we noticed a poster advertising an open air Rolling Stones concert at the Sydney Cricket Ground (SCG). The tickets cost as many dollars as we had budgeted to last for about five days, but we all agreed it would be an unforgettable experience and we'd treat ourselves and go. We weren't disappointed—the concert was absolutely brilliant. That was my first time at the SCG. Little did I know I'd be spending quite a bit of time there in the not too distant future.

We began our adventure by catching a Greyhound bus up the east coast, stopping off at Byron Bay, Airlie Beach, Fraser Island (where we camped out and I saw my first dingo) and the Whitsunday Islands—all of it absolutely beautiful. In Cairns, we booked to go on a boat trip out to the Barrier Reef. It was to be one of the highlights of our visit. The boat was a sailing boat big enough to accommodate ten people together with three crew: captain, cook and deckhand. We were all very excited about our trip out to the reef—it's an experience a lot of people can only dream about. The trip out to the reef would take about three hours then we would weigh anchor overnight and go snorkelling the next day. Unfortunately for us, this was the time when cyclone Agnes was hitting that area of Australia's coastline. Not being a particularly strong swimmer and having a fear of deep water, I was a little apprehensive, to say the least, about the prospect of sailing out into the wide blue yonder in cyclone conditions. The Captain, Paul, informed us that the cyclone was quite a way from us and that although the conditions might be a bit rough, we'd be fine. We all frantically downed our Kwells and tried to prepare ourselves for the journey. As we approached Green Island, the last piece of land before the reef, the sea had become extremely rough and a few of us—well, mainly me— were becoming a little concerned. Paul called a meeting and told us that the boat could handle these weather conditions; the question was, could we? There was a unanimous decision to continue, so on we went. 'A bit rough', the Captain had said. The ocean was like a huge, green, wobbly jelly rollercoaster and I was convinced we were all going to die. Really! You know when you're so frightened you start laughing hysterically? I was at that stage, clinging on to the roof of the cabin for dear life. Well, we made it out to the reef, safe and sound and, miraculously, none the worse for our epic journey. Mind you, there was still the sail back to Cairns to go. The Kwells had been marvellous. The snorkelling was amazing and well worth the trip, however terrifying it had been. It was most definitely a character-building voyage.

My first trip Down Under proved to be an unforgettable experience and I fell in love with Australia. It was the country with everything: fantastic beaches, tropical rainforests, endless sunshine, wide open spaces, fascinating wildlife—what more could anyone ask for?

IN THE BEGINNING

My work friend Karen and I loved going to Hong Kong (Honkers, as we affectionately called it) and had requested a trip together. Her divorce had just been granted and she was keen to go out and celebrate—the nightlife in Hong Kong can be pretty lively, so that's where we decided to go. There was a bit of a glitch in our plans when we received our monthly rosters and discovered that she had been allocated the trip and I hadn't. However, I had been put on standby that day, and as luck or fate would have it, one of the crew went sick and I was called out in her place.

Virgin's Hong Kong trips were all two-nighters. With the time difference between Hong Kong and London being eight hours, this made it perfect for us to go out all night and sleep during the day. Quite often, we'd be returning to our hotel after a night out and see the local children going to school. Our system actually worked very well—our return flight to London was an evening departure, so after having slept for most of the day, we'd take off from Hong Kong feeling refreshed and more than ready to cope with the demands of the twelve-hour flight back home.

On this particular occasion, having been out to a couple of clubs on the first night, I wasn't all that keen to go out and do it again the following night. Karen was extremely disappointed and begged me to change my mind and go out with her; we were here to have fun and had requested the trip especially after all. I eventually succumbed to her powers of persuasion and agreed to go but told her that I couldn't be bothered to make any special effort—wash my hair, do my nails or dress up—I'd go as I was, like it or not. I hoped this might put her off, but she wasn't to be deterred. We were going out on the town and that was that. Little did I know I was about to meet the man of my dreams and future husband. Mind you, had I known, I'd probably have been too nervous to go out at all! A couple of our flight deck crew came out with us—they were always great chaperones. Our hotel was situated on the mainland, which meant we had to catch a taxi through the tunnel and across to Hong Kong island, which took about twenty minutes. We went to one of our favourite haunts; a club called Joe Bananas (JBs) in Wan Chai, the area of Hong Kong where most of the bars and nightclubs can be found. When we arrived, there were quite a few people in the club but it wasn't unbearable. I hate it when the room gets so crowded you can't move, or get to the bar. Karen and I went off to the Ladies (as girls do, in pairs) and when we returned and made our way to the bar, Graham, one of our flight deck chaperones, informed us that several members of the Australian cricket team were in the club and had asked to meet us. Graham had been known to pull our legs once or twice in the past, and thinking this was another of his jokes, our response was 'sure, send them over'. I think we were both quite shocked when Graham turned and gave a couple of lads the nod and over they came and introduced themselves. They weren't a bad-looking bunch, and I was beginning to feel quite glad Karen had talked me into coming out. Glenn was the last one to introduce himself, which made me think he wasn't particularly interested. Karen soon disappeared off onto the dance floor leaving me with the others, our flight crew watching from a discreet distance. Glenn offered to buy me a drink, which is always a good start, and it wasn't long before we were chatting away and getting on like a house on fire. I liked him instantly. He was really easy to talk to, very down-to-earth and funny, not to mention particularly easy on the eye! I asked him about Australia and told him about my backpacking adventure, at the back of my mind thinking what a shame it was that he lived so far away and I'd probably never see him again. I asked what had brought him to Honkers. He

IN THE BEGINNING

explained that they were there for a few days to take part in a cricket sixes competition and that they were actually playing the following day. Unfortunately, Karen and I were unable to go and watch the match as we were leaving for Heathrow later that same day, which was a bit disappointing. Glenn and I ended our evening by exchanging phone numbers and addresses and that was that. He walked off in one direction and I went in the other, thinking again what a pity it was that he couldn't have lived just a little bit closer.

I discovered the next day that they'd lost their game. This didn't come as a huge surprise—after JBs, we'd all gone to a dance club across the road and we hadn't left until about 3.30 am.

The next evening flying home to London (which is an awfully long way from Sydney), I couldn't stop thinking about Glenn. Although I couldn't quite put my finger on it, I knew there was something very special about him. After we'd completed the meal service, there was time for Karen and I to sit down and have a cup of tea and a chat. We'd had a terrific time in Hong Kong, and I thanked her for persuading me to go out. I asked her if she felt that there had been something really special about the previous evening, because that was how I felt but I didn't really know why. 'It was fun,' she laughed, 'but we always have a good time there.'

To me, for some inexplicable reason, my evening at JBs hadn't felt like any other I'd spent there. I wondered if I'd get to see Glenn again or if that one night in Hong Kong would be the first and last we'd ever share together.

G Unlike Jane, I've been a loner since I was young. While many of the blokes I grew up with stuck together in packs, chased girls and made beelines to the local watering holes once they turned eighteen, I enjoyed my own company.

Local folklore suggests that Australia's great bush balladist Banjo Paterson—the author of *Waltzing Matilda*, *The Man From Ironbark* and *Clancy of the Overflow*—passed through Narromine during his travels in the late 19th century, and I'm certain he would have been moved by the same sights and sounds which made an impression on me: the sulphur-crested cockatoos, timid kangaroos, flocks of galahs at sunset, angry-looking emus and the everlasting glory of the Far West's night sky. While I could never hope to describe the beauty of the country with Banjo's flair, I often find that when I'm away on tour with the Aussie cricket team, or even at home in Sydney, my thoughts wander back to the bush tracks and sunlit plains of my childhood and I sometimes feel a longing to go bush and escape. I can't help that feeling—it's in my blood. My parents, their parents and, I think, their folks are sons and daughters of the outback. They've lived through drought, flood, depression, world wars, stock losses, crippling bank interest rates and failed crops. Their experiences have made them hardy and proud people, and I like to think I've inherited some of their fighting qualities.

While I'm proud to call Narromine home, I was actually born in Dubbo, the Far West's major town and Australia's fastest growing inland city. My formative years were spent there on our family's poultry farm, where my grandparents, mother, father, uncles and aunts ran the whole shebang. We moved to the Lagoona property outside Narromine when I turned three. For a number of years Mum and Dad battled a litany of disasters to try and make a fist of their lot. It was an unforgiving lifestyle and I quickly learned the value of hard work—bloody hard work—by slaving out in the fields. Indeed, I reckon I scrubbed at least an acre's worth of dirt from under

IN THE BEGINNING

my fingernails during my teenage years. One tough time tattooed on my mind is when my brother Dale and I were assigned the task of sowing 243 hectares of crops while our father was in the Northern Territory trying to make some extra dollars. It was a case of two boys attempting to do a man's job, and, even today, a lifetime later, I can vividly recall the exhaustion I felt at the end of each eleven-hour shift. Nothing I have done since then—even bowling marathon spells on flat tracks in India—has matched that feeling of mind-numbing tiredness.

Nevertheless, I have mainly happy memories of Lagoona. I still smile when I recall the backyard Tests Dale, my sister Donna and I played behind Dad's workshop.

Rather than chase the so-called 'bright lights', I would wander deep into the bush which surrounded our property to hunt wild pigs, feral goats and the cunning foxes which sometimes raided our chicken coops when we were asleep. I still enjoy the thrill of the hunt, because there's a sense of adventure to it, and when I reflect upon my childhood, it feels as if I was never as carefree—or alive—as when I was out among the ghost gums and the wild scrub. People immediately think the worst when they hear I have a penchant for hunting—I can see it in their eyes—but I do respect life. You see, pulling the trigger is only one per cent of the experience. For instance, there have been many times when I have stalked a couple of porkers . . . crept right up on them . . . and then followed my footsteps back through the scrub without them knowing I'd been among them. For me, that's the thrill of the hunt.

When I was about fifteen my parents' marriage broke up. I think my brother and sister were more affected by the split than me because I was older, more independent, and I had my sport and other interests to take my mind off things. I also viewed their divorce from a different angle. In an ideal world families would stay together and they wouldn't argue or fight, but when the reality of a relationship is constant fighting and bickering, the people involved have to ask whether there is any point—or benefit—in staying together. Most often there's not. Regardless, both Mum and Dad made sure we felt loved and secure.

While I enjoyed maths and science at school, I was far from the greatest scholar to leave the gates of Narromine High School... though I was also far from the worst. Most of my time away from the classroom was spent playing basketball, competition golf or cricket, or hunting wild pigs with razor-sharp tusks. But nothing appealed to me quite like cricket. It is well documented that during my youth few people—if any—thought I had any cricketing ability. However, I had an unshakeable belief I would one day open the bowling for the Australian Test side. The image of me bowling in a Test was so real I sometimes had to pinch myself to see if it was happening. While most of my mates were well aware that I bowled at a rusty old 44-gallon-drum for hours at a time, I didn't dare to tell them about my dream. I kept that a secret because I feared being ridiculed. You see, while I was dreaming of partnering Dennis Lillee and Craig McDermott in the Australian side, I wasn't even considered good enough to bowl for my under-16 team, the Backwater XI! My skipper, Shane Horsborough, dismissed me as nothing more than a kid who helped make up the numbers each weekend, and he kept me hidden from the action by making me patrol the outfield. Many of my friends thought I would have been better off concentrating on basketball after I was selected to represent the Far West in the burgeoning State League competition. It was a hoot, but the American game didn't grab me the way cricket did... I was more interested in following in the footsteps of Ray Lindwall, Jeff Thomson and Lillee than those of Wilt Chamberlain and Michael Jordan.

IN THE BEGINNING

Though I did well at basketball and golf, cricket was my first love and I spent hours bowling out some of the world's best batsmen of that era—Desmond Haynes, Viv Richards, Martin Crowe, David Gower and the big-hitting Brit Ian Botham. On such occasions the bumpy pitch behind Dad's workshop suddenly transformed into the Sydney Cricket Ground and I pictured myself running in at them from the Randwick end and letting rip with a fireball to the wild cheers of the mob on the hill. It may only have been a kid's fantasy, but my belief even then was that if you're going to dream, you might as well reach for the stars. It was sometimes hard, but I didn't allow the lack of interest shown in me by the people at Backwater to deter me. I just kept plugging away until one day it fell into place and a few people suddenly saw the traits I'd always possessed. Some described my success on the local cricket pitches as an overnight miracle, but I can assure you there's an old, dented, twisted, rust-eaten 44-gallon-tin crushed beneath a mountain of rubbish in the Narromine tip which tells the real story. Practice and faith.

While I firmly believed I would one day make it as a cricketer, I also made plans to make an income outside of the game—just in case. I left school when I completed my Year 10 School Certificate, and armed with that I enrolled in the carpentry course at Tech. I wanted to be a builder, to do something with my hands. One very enjoyable part of my course was helping to build two houses which the Tech sold to make extra money. It was a wonderful experience, and I guess my class did something right because almost fourteen years down the track they're still standing and looking solid.

Unfortunately, as is often the way in the outback, there were no jobs available when I finished the course so I was forced to do labouring work and that was hard bloody yakka. I ploughed paddocks, built and repaired fences, bent my back in our neighbour's cotton fields and did lots of other manual work. Sometimes I slaved up to 70 hours a week, and while I might not have necessarily enjoyed the work, it was certainly a lot better than being on the dole. The labouring could be lucrative, too. After a few months I saved enough cash to buy a Holden Commodore, and for a while it was my pride and joy. But I knew that labouring was limited as far as job opportunities were concerned, and when I later landed a job with the State Bank I knew it was a step in the right direction. For a start the office was airconditioned. And rather than a 'flanny' and weatherbeaten Akubra, I wore a collar and tie.

As I've said, I'm proud to call Narromine my home and have loved the bush from an early age, but I also wanted to travel and see the world. I'd study maps and atlases for hours at a time. I wanted to meet people . . . I wanted to experience life and I desired new challenges. I also thought it would be something to meet a decent girl to share it all with. I didn't have a girlfriend when I was growing up in Narromine—I was shy, and I was happy to be a loner.

In the end, cricket was my ticket out. While Mum and Dad are adamant my sister Donna was the standout bowler in our backyard Tests (I trust they're only kidding!), I was eventually selected, at the age of eighteen, in the Dubbo representative side which played Parkes in a Toohey's Country Cup match. The Country Cup was an initiative (and a brilliant one) to take First Class players such as Doug Walters, Steve and Mark Waugh, Mark Taylor, Steve Small, Graeme Beard, Mike Whitney and Dirk Wellham to the outback and pit them against us bush-bashers. It was as much about allowing outback supporters to see the stars as it was about giving the 'hayseeds' their shot. Indeed, I have no hesitation in nominating that game at Parkes as being my big break. I was up against then aspiring Test batsman Mark Waugh and the hero

IN THE BEGINNING

of the old SCG Hill, Kevin Douglas 'Doug' Walters. The Dubbo team was galvanised by the inclusion of future Test skipper Mark Taylor and then Test all-rounder Greg Matthews.

Walters was at the crease when I was given the ball as Dubbo's first change bowler. The wind was knocked out of my sails somewhat when Matthews advised me to show Doug the respect he deserved. Greg didn't need to do that . . . I had far too much time for Doug's achievements to try anything too brazen. Firstly, Walters was two years into his retirement and secondly, when he put the last of his First Class caps into mothballs he did so with a Test batting average of 48.26 and a highest score of 250. While I wanted to dismiss him because of his reputation, I had no intention of being a smart alec. Instead, I planned to simply bowl a nice, tight line to him. My plan was almost rewarded when he popped a catch to one of our close-in fieldsmen. Unfortunately it was too hot to handle, and I missed out on his prized scalp. Then, as if to rub salt into my wounds, I was denied a hat-trick (three wickets in three balls) when two more catches slipped through my team-mates' fingers. It was one heck of an experience, but when I returned home to a cup of cocoa with Mum and Dad I dismissed the match as one of those 'what should've been' moments and prepared to get back on with life at the Bank.

Unbeknownst to me Doug had made a mental note of my name, and on his return to Sydney he phoned Steve Rixon, the then NSW Sheffield Shield side's coach, and gave me an almighty wrap. It was on Doug's recommendation that Steve phoned to invite me to join his grade club, Sutherland, in Sydney. It was a dream come true, and felt even more special because it came from out of the blue. Actually, I feared I'd already missed my chance of playing in Sydney: only a few weeks before Rixon's phone call another club, Penrith, had dispatched a talent scout to see if I could cut the mustard. He thought not. After watching me bowl he put a thick red line through my name, and I'm willing to bet he dismissed the 400-odd kilometre journey over the Blue Mountains as a complete waste of time. The poor bugger probably cursed me all the way home.

While we live in the age of telecommunications, and the Internet and email are making the world a lot smaller, I don't think anything quite matches the speed of the ol' bush telegraph for spreading news. It didn't take long for my offer from Sutherland to become public knowledge. While most of the folk in Narromine were ecstatic for me, there were one or two sadsacks who said I was only setting myself up to be ripped to pieces... they figured I was better off staying in the bush. I should note that the same people said something similar when David Gillespie left home to play for the Canterbury Rugby League side in the old Winfield Cup competition and when Melinda Gainsford-Taylor took her first steps towards running at the Olympics. Anyway, I took no notice of them. I was too excited to entertain any negative vibes and, anyway, I had Mum's positive energy to draw from—she said it was a great opportunity and I had to embrace the move for all it was worth.

Dad was happy for me, but Dad is a man of the bush. While he was extremely proud of the opportunity then and is even more proud of my achievements since, he really can't relate to my life as a professional sportsman. He is more in tune with the ways of my brother Dale, who has stayed on the land, and I accept that.

When Dale isn't tending to the livestock or crops he does things like drive road trains to the Top End, and while I spend hours analysing the batting styles of such opponents as West Indies batsman Brian Lara and India's Sachin Tendulkar, Dale and Dad watch the weather with a mind as to how it will affect their crops, and, ultimately, their income. Nevertheless, Dad has made numerous trips to watch me play at the SCG — but I believe his personal highlight from spending time in the stands was the night he met television personality Kerri-Anne Kennerley!

Mum went way above the call of duty when she volunteered to tow the caravan which was to be my new Sydney home (it was more affordable than renting an apartment) to the big smoke because she knew the city much better than me. I left Narromine at a breakneck pace and in a cloud of dust, but Mum actually beat me to the caravan park. I must admit I felt like a bit of a kid when Mum prepared to leave the following day; I wasn't properly prepared to leave a huge property — and loving family — to live in a tin shoebox on wheels. Indeed, Mum later told me it was hard for her not to cave into the motherly instinct to turn around and give me a big hug and say everything would be alright.

There weren't too many wild nights out on the town during my first few months in Sydney. While I made some firm friendships among my new team-mates, my schedule was totally regimented: I'd wake up; eat breakfast; shower and shave; work at the State Bank; eat lunch; return to the caravan; train; walk along Ramsgate Beach; have dinner; watch television; iron my work gear; hit the sack. I followed that routine for thirteen long months. However, I wasn't in the Harbour City to be a social butterfly . . . I was there to earn my stripes as a fast bowler. And not just any fast bowler. I wanted to play Test cricket for the world's greatest team.

I don't mind conceding it could be bloody boring waiting for my destiny to be fulfilled. I spent a lot of my time in the caravan dreaming about that baggy green cap . . . and I thought a lot about many other things. Things like where I hoped to be in a decade's time, the woman I hoped to one day settle down with, the countries I wanted to visit and experiences I hoped to savour. But the Test cricket cap was the lure which drove me most of all.

While I had always believed I would one day make the Australian team, I have to admit it was one hell of a shock when I was given my call-to-arms in the national team to play against New Zealand in the first Test match in Perth. The critics described it as a rapid rise through the ranks because I'd only played a handful of Sheffield Shield games for the Blues. Nevertheless, I walked on air for a week.

If I say it once, I'll say it a million times; one of the great advantages of being an international sportsman is the opportunity it provides to tour foreign countries; sometimes when the team is jetting its way to yet another nation for another series I feel as though I really have been blessed. As a kid it was always my dream to play for Australia and to see the world— and I have managed to achieve both by being able to hurl a cricket ball at 130-odd kilometres an hour. You sometimes hear athletes moaning about the amount of touring and time away from home they're forced to endure. I can't help but shake my head in disbelief. You see, I take none of it for granted because I know the time will come when it all ends—and no one knows when that might happen. That's why I make a point of taking time out whenever I'm in a foreign land to try and absorb some of the local culture. While it is more often than not just a matter of scratching the surface—like visiting a bazaar in dusty Lahore, going on a short safari in South Africa or riding an elephant in the Highlands of Sri Lanka—I at least make the effort.

Sometimes, in a place such as India, it can be very hard to

IN THE BEGINNING

get a glimpse of everyday life because a player can quite easily become the pied piper of Mumbai or Calcutta by venturing out on the streets. Believe me, literally hundreds of people follow your every step and watch your every move. The locals not only love their cricket, but they also idolise the players with a fervour unsurpassed in any other nation. Sometimes their reaction to being up-close-and-personal can be quite humbling, if not downright embarrassing: some of the Indians who have mobbed me knew more about me than I did. It floored me to learn some of them even knew the name of the property I grew up on at Narromine: La-bloody-goona!

However, there are also occasions when we lob at a place such as Hong Kong or Dubai and the locals don't know us from a bar of soap. In 1995, after my first matches playing for Australia I found myself in Hong Kong to compete in a Sixes tournament at the Koowloon Cricket Club. We had just completed a historic triumph in the Caribbean—a rare Test series victory over the Windies on their home soil—and we were in the mood to celebrate.

I was certainly in the mood, given that the tour of the Caribbean marked my coming of age as a Test cricketer. A serious injury to our key bowler Craig McDermott presented me with the golden opportunity and I grabbed it. I finished the series with the most Australian wickets, seventeen, and a few man-of-the-match awards, and I celebrated my success with a litre or two of the local rum. The series also instilled a real sense of confidence in me—the added responsibility made me feel that I really was a member of the Australian team.

Well, the heavy hangover from the rum accompanied me to the old British colony of Hong Kong, where we were asked to fly cricket's flag in the Sixes tournament—a condensed version of the one day game. The Sixes was formulated as part of the International Cricket Council's attempt to make inroads into

Asia. I guess the powers that be were inspired by Rugby Union's immense success with the Hong Kong Sevens. The Sevens not only attracts some of that sport's biggest names, but it also commands worldwide media attention and huge sponsorship dollars. While the hospitality for us flannelled fools was warm, the interest in the cricket was a distant cry from the buzz which accompanies the Rugby festival. Nevertheless, Michael Slater, Greg Blewett, Brendon Julian, Matthew Hayden, Matt Elliott and I were entrusted with the duty of doing Australia proud but to be brutally honest, we put far greater effort into enjoying the nightlife of Hong Kong than we did into hitting the white ball for six. We enjoyed one victory but I think South Africa won the trophy. They had a deadly serious attitude and enforced strict curfews, drinking bans and the like.

We Aussies had no such restrictions. The highlight of our nocturnal adventures was the night a few of us spent on Nathan Road, aka The Golden Mile. If I'd known I was about to meet the great love of my life, I would have probably been a lot more nervous than I was. First stop was a night club called Joe Bananas; the supposed promised land for red-blooded blokes in Hong Kong. I was told it was a popular hangout for flight crews, and from all reports it was a good place to relax and unwind. However, once we arrived I saw it was just like any nightclub anywhere in the world.

What did make it different, though, was one of the air hostesses there . . . she was tall, blonde, bright-eyed and always smiling; a bloke would have had to have been as dull as a fishing pole not to have noticed her. One of our group, I think it might have been Brendon Julian (he's reputed to be a bit of a charmer), made the first brave step towards her group. The girls were happy to chat. It didn't take long for us to realise that they too were out to enjoy themselves. Karen was 'celebrating' her divorce, while the smiling one, Jane, was there to simply enjoy the party.

If it is possible to be captivated by a complete stranger, then I was—hook, line and sinker. Jane Steele had a vibrant personality—brighter even than the millions of tiny coloured lights in Kowloon—and she lit the poky nightclub up when she smiled. Oh, and she knew absolutely nothing about cricket. After a few drinks—and many more laughs—we moved on to another nightclub which had been recommended by a few people, but it was a dump. There were seedy types propped up against the bar; the drinks were expensive; the music was dreadful and it was dingy with a capital 'D'. However, in terms of the night it didn't matter—I could have been in a Chinese laundry with my new English chum watching old t-shirts spin around in a drier and it would probably have still been fun. The time—all twelve hours—flew by too quickly, and like Cinderella returning home from the ball Jane hitched a ride in a cab with a couple of fair dinkum Aussie pumpkins: Brendon and me. One thing I can vividly recall about that cab trip, apart from the crazy driver who wouldn't have even been allowed on a dodgem car back in Sydney, is Jane's infamous watermelon joke. You don't want to know it, it's ordinary and you need to see her hand signals to appreciate it. However, it is also rather risqué, and I couldn't help but notice Jane blushed like an over-ripe tomato after she told it. It was almost is if she couldn't believe she had said it. Not that it mattered—despite her poor idea of a joke I was still attracted to her.

While I was being sincere when I promised to keep in touch after we exchanged our details, I have to admit that at that stage of my life I was very much the single man about town, and I was out to seize the moment and to enjoy myself. After all, I was living every young bloke's dream . . . travelling the world with a high-profile sporting side and enjoying most of the fringe benefits. But, I guess you can't escape destiny, and while I didn't quite hear it at the time, I'm sure there must have been a whisper deep within my mind saying Jane was someone special ... A few hours after Jane and I said our farewells my team-mates and I attended a coaching clinic for the colony's young cricketers. For all I know there may have been a budding Don Bradman or Dennis Lillee among the many keen, smiling faces but I was heavy-eyed and tired. While I told the kids everything I thought was worthwhile I was working overtime to stifle my yawns. And yes, while showing the future of Hong Kong cricket the best grips to employ when bowling off-cutters and bouncers I spared a thought or two for Jane. However, she had gone her way and I had gone mine — I didn't even know if our paths would ever cross again.

LOVE BLOSSOMS

J Following our trip to Honkers, I'd been home for about a week, feeling a bit flat, when I remembered I'd booked a week's leave at the beginning of December 1995. I decided to write to Glenn, casually mentioning the fact that I could pop out to Sydney to see him if he wasn't doing anything. A bit forward I know, but there was no harm in asking. I didn't know at this point that he played Test cricket for Australia (I wouldn't have understood what that meant had he told me), let alone anything about how hectic the cricket season actually is. Anyway, three weeks passed and I heard nothing. A little disappointed, I decided that that was that, he obviously wasn't interested. It had just been a flash in the pan. Then very early one morning in November, I returned from a Miami trip to my little Cotswold cottage, absolutely shattered after the flight and the three-hour drive home from Gatwick airport, poured myself a cup of Earl Grey tea and played back my answering machine messages. And there it was, at last—a message from Glenn. I could not believe my ears—he'd called! What I really couldn't believe was that he'd called and I hadn't been there. Typical. I must have played that message back a hundred times, with a smile from ear to ear. I was flying to Tokyo later that week so I thought I'd wait and call him from there, as the time difference wasn't as great. And more to the point, I didn't want to appear too keen. After all, he'd kept me waiting three weeks, the cheeky devil! However, when I called him back from Tokyo, it was my turn to leave a message, as this time he was away. I left my hotel number for him and went out with the crew, not really expecting him to call straight away—it'd probably take him at least another three weeks. When I returned from my evening out (we'd been in a karaoke bar) there was a message waiting for me—Glenn had rung. I was surprised and thrilled. I dashed to my room and returned his call straight away, not wanting to miss him again and, what do you know, he actually answered the phone. He told me he'd received my letter, but during the time of my leave, he'd be playing in a Test match in Perth against Sri Lanka. I immediately wished I'd never sent it. Then he asked if I'd like to fly over and stay with him to watch the game. I nearly fell over. I'd never been to Perth or watched a Test match so I said yes, my heart racing. I went to sleep feeling very pleased with myself.

As I knew nothing whatsoever about the game of cricket, one of the first things I did when I got back home to Little Compton was to go out to Stratford-on-Avon to search for a book on cricket. I eventually settled on *The Rules and Regulations of Cricket*. It appeared to be able to tell me everything I needed to know—if I was going to sit and watch cricket for five days, I wanted to understand what the game was all about (mind you, sometimes I'm still not sure).

My Dad wasn't very impressed at my flying out to Australia for a week. I think maybe he felt that Glenn should be the one jetting over to England to see me, not vice versa.

I had mentioned Glenn's name to him but Dad hadn't heard of him.

As departure day drew nearer, I was both excited and apprehensive. Finally I was almost there. The Virgin crew on my flight were lovely, and I was allocated a seat in Upper Class (Virgin's name for their Business Class section). It wasn't until I was actually sitting back in my seat, sipping my glass of chilled champagne and taxiing down the runway, that I began to wonder what on earth I was doing. I began to think I must have lost my marbles. Here I was, with a week off work, flying to the other side of the world to Australia to meet a man I'd only spent a few hours with and watch a game I knew absolutely nothing about. Had I completely lost the plot? All I knew was that I had no control over it. Sanity and commonsense had gone out of the window and in their place was something much bigger—I simply had to go, and that was that. There was no choice. And if the worst came to the worst and he turned out to be an axe murderer or psycho or just a pain in the bottom, then I'd simply fly back home. No problem.

It wasn't until I finally arrived in Perth, about twenty-four hours later, that I seriously started to get cold feet. I very nearly got on the next plane back to London without even leaving the airport. Whilst waiting for my suitcase to appear on the luggage carousel, I popped into the Ladies to compose myself. I eventually managed to pull myself together, grabbed my bag, caught a taxi and went off to the Hyatt, where the team was staying. Due to an afternoon training session, Glenn had been unable to meet me at the airport, which was probably a blessing, as I'd got myself into such a state. I tried to focus on my new surroundings and how beautiful the weather was, but to no avail. By the time the taxi pulled up at the front of the Hyatt, about twenty minutes later, I felt like an absolute wreck, exhausted and extremely nervous. The bellboy came out to help me with my luggage and I explained I was here to see one of the guests. He directed me over to the house phone, where I called Glenn, who gave me his room number and told me to come up. He didn't even ask if I needed any help with my bags. Not very chivalrous after I'd flown round the world to see him, I thought to myself. I staggered along the hallway to his room—which, of course, was right at the end—dragging my suitcase behind me. I was practically on my knees I was so tired. I took a deep breath and nervously knocked on the door. I was feeling extremely self-conscious by this stage, and when Glenn answered the door, I managed to blurt out a quick 'Hello' before walking into the room rather hurriedly with my head down, wishing I looked a little more glamorous. He was even more handsome than I'd remembered and I was instantly glad I'd made the journey. He poured me a cool drink and we chatted until I nodded off, which wasn't long—he must have been impressed!

The following day was the first day of the Test and Glenn was up and out early, leaving me for a very welcome lie-in. He'd left me a ticket at the Members' Gate at the Western Australian Cricket Association ground, the WACA. I turned up at the ground at about 2.30 pm, not realising the day's play had already started. My little book hadn't mentioned that. As I walked into the ground I could see from the scoreboard that Australia were fielding. It looked like Glenn bowling but I wasn't sure. There were quite a few people around so I asked one of them who the bowler was. 'That's Glenn McGrath' came the reply. Great timing, I thought, very pleased with myself.

It was an absolutely beautiful day, warm and sunny and not a cloud in the sky. I found myself beginning to understand why people feel the need to take all their clothes off and go streaking across that lush green cricket pitch! Hastily, I bought myself a drink, found a seat and settled down to watch my first cricket session. I'd taken my rulebook with me just in case. I had a great afternoon, and decided I'd aim to be there a little bit earlier the next day.

During the evenings we'd go out to dinner or to the casino. On one occasion, the boys had been invited to a Joshua Kadison concert. He sings and plays the piano, a bit like Elton John but younger, and Glenn asked me if I'd like to go. I'd never heard of 'Jason Cassidy' (which was what I thought Glenn had said), but as I love live music, I agreed to go along. He had arranged to meet the other boys down in the bar and took me down there with him. I decided at this point that I didn't want to go after all—I didn't want to meet the others and be scrutinised. It was all too nerve-racking. Glenn assured me they wouldn't bite, so off I went, reluctantly. When we walked into the bar, I could see some of the boys sitting down at a long table. A few others were standing up. Amazingly, there were no other girls around. We walked in, me feeling extremely self-conscious and praying I wouldn't go over on my ankle or trip up. I hid behind Glenn as he got me a drink at the bar and then, horror of horrors, one of the boys called him over to their table and he left me with the group standing at the bar. I nearly died. Should I follow him or stay where I was? I ended up staying where I was, doing my best to look as if I couldn't have cared less. I was relieved when an older man in the group turned round and started chatting to me. He'd been to England a couple of times so we talked about that. He seemed really quite nice. I was wondering whose dad he might be and was about to ask him that very question when Glenn called me over to the table as everyone was getting ready to leave for the concert. As we walked out to the taxis, I told Glenn I'd been chatting to an older man who was with them and was really nice. I asked Glenn who had their dad with them, as I couldn't recall him telling me his name. Glenn laughed and told me that the man I'd been talking to was actually the team coach, Bob Simpson. I was very relieved I hadn't asked him who his son was!

Australia ended up winning the Test, beating Sri Lanka by an innings and 36 runs, with Glenn taking seven wickets for the match. I flew back to Sydney with him and we spent a couple of days together at his flat in Cronulla, which had a definite bachelor pad feel about it. I loved Cronulla. It had a really good, relaxed atmosphere. The golden beaches and the sparkling ocean were just beautiful, and I could easily see why he'd chosen to live there. There were some great little cafes and restaurants but not loads of tourists or crowds. I was having an absolutely wonderful time. I'd really enjoyed my first Test match and Glenn had been great company. Too soon it was time to head back to London. I thanked Glenn for a lovely trip, but decided not to say too much more. I knew he was happy with his single life and not looking for a relationship. I had taken a little Christmas present with me for him but I decided against giving it to him. I got the distinct impression I wasn't the only woman in his life and I wasn't about to let him think that I cared too much. Cricket was most definitely his priority; he'd made that very clear.

Despite the fact that I'd seen Glenn playing in a Test match, I had never seen a one day game. I had a trip to San Francisco on New Year's Day 1996 and decided to give him a quick call from there to wish him a Happy New Year. Unbeknownst to me, it had been the day of that one-dayer against the West Indies, when Australia needed five runs to win the game and Glenn came in midway through the final over to join Michael Bevan at the crease. I've seen that game since on video and can barely watch it even now without feeling excited and nervous—despite knowing the outcome. Anyway, I asked Glenn what kind of a day he'd had and he began telling me about the game. He described in great detail how tremendously exciting the final over had been and that he'd hit a single and put Michael on strike and Michael had hit a four off the last ball and Australia had won. But it was all totally lost on me at the time—he may as well have been speaking in a foreign language. I didn't have a clue what he was talking about so I just said something like 'really, oh that's good then, that you won', and changed the subject. Now I know he'd just played in one of the most memorable and exciting one day games ever.

Following that trip to Perth, Glenn and I were ringing each other every week or so, and it was during one of these calls that he asked me if I'd like to go back out to Sydney for a holiday, maybe for a month or two.

After the success of my backpacking expedition Down Under, I'd already booked two months' unpaid leave from Virgin for April and May, with a view to doing something similar, maybe in New Zealand this time. But I found the prospect of spending a month with Glenn infinitely more exciting and so it was all arranged. I would fly out to Australia in April for a month or so and we'd see how we got on. I was very excited, but also aware that being with the same person for a month or two under the same roof would be a real test, and it may not be all smooth sailing. If that was the case, I would just fly home or else go off and do some exploring by myself.

This time Glenn was there to meet me at Sydney airport, albeit a little late (he remembers this differently!). His grade team, Sutherland, had beaten Bankstown (Mark and Steve Waugh's team) and won the Premiership the day before I arrived and the boys had been out doing some serious celebrating. Needless to say, he was a little worse for wear. It was still great to see him again.

During my stay, Glenn suggested we take a holiday. He had already been to the travel agent and got lots of brochures. After thumbing through them, we decided on a beautiful resort up on the edge of the rainforest just north of Cairns. The resort, Bloomfield, was quite exclusive and accessible only by boat, so getting there was an adventure in itself. We flew to Cairns and overnighted there in a hotel, catching a flight in a light aircraft the following morning. I hadn't realised how casual life is over here and as I knew Bloomfield was quite a select resort, I'd packed a couple of evening dresses that I'd brought with me together with strappy shoes and all the little extras. When we came to board the light plane, my bag was way too heavy and they told me I'd have to leave some things behind. Much to my embarrassment, I had to sift through its contents, deciding what was necessary and what wasn't with Glenn looking on, commenting and laughing at all the dressy things I'd brought with me on a trip to the rainforest. Needless to say, we left most of my belongings behind in Cairns.

The short, spectacular flight to Bloomfield took us out along the coastline and over the ocean, then back inland over rainforest and a wonderful waterfall before we landed at last on a very bumpy grass airstrip. From there, we were taken by four-wheel drive to a mooring on the Bloomfield River, where a smallish boat was waiting to transport us to the resort. Glenn had booked us into the honeymoon cabin (I think by mistake!) and so during our entire week's stay, the staff referred to us as Mr and Mrs McGrath, which we found quite amusing though we were a little taken aback at first. We didn't bother setting people straight, just said, 'Oh, call us Glenn and Jane.' One evening, I remember sitting around the pool area before dinner sipping cocktails when an older couple joined us for a drink. They assumed we were girlfriend and boyfriend, and asked how long we'd been together. 'Oh no, she's not my girlfriend,' came Glenn's reply, quick as a flash, 'Jane's just a friend over from England. We've come up here for a little break, that's all.' I wanted the ground to open up and swallow me. I was absolutely gutted. We'd gone from being Mr and Mrs McGrath to him making me feel like his latest tart and passing me off as no one special in front of complete strangers whose opinion should have meant nothing to him anyway. I didn't know whether to crawl under the table with humiliation or smack him across the face! As it was I just sat there, putting on a brave face and laughing it off, but I was hurting inside. By this time, I was beginning to fall for him, and had considered telling him how I felt. Now it was only too painfully clear how he felt, and if I could have left and flown home right there and then, I would have. (I delight in reminding him of that moment now—he can't believe he was so insensitive and hurtful.) After that night at least I knew where I stood. I decided to simply enjoy myself and Glenn's company for what it was, and expect nothing more.

There was no television and no newspapers at the resort, but we found that we didn't miss them at all. We went for walks through the rainforest where I saw spider webs the size of tennis courts—you can imagine the size of the spiders! We went snorkelling out on the Barrier Reef and learnt to scuba dive. We took a picnic out to the rocks by the water's edge and watched the huge turtles swimming by. Glenn went fishing off the jetty most evenings but would get cross if there was anyone else down there who didn't really know what they were doing. He gets like that when he's playing blackjack too. Each evening at about six pm, we'd wander down to the honour bar and he'd create various cocktails and then we'd sit around and talk and eat dinner. It was a great getaway, and so relaxing.

Apart from his comment at dinner that night, our time at the Bloomfield resort was wonderful. It wasn't until we were on our way home that we realised just how cut off we'd been. We were sitting in the Gold Wing lounge at Cairns airport waiting for our connecting flight back to Sydney when we read in the newspapers about the terrible massacre down in Port Arthur and were totally shocked, both that it had happened and that we had known nothing about it.

One of the highlights of my stay in Sydney was being able to go to the weddings of two of Glenn's friends. One was Neil and Kate Maxwell's wedding. Neil and Kate had their wedding reception at Taronga Zoo. Part of the package was that the Zoo lets you choose an animal for your guests to see and meet when they first arrive at the reception. Neil and Kate had chosen a baby wombat. On arriving at the reception, I had popped into the loo, and when I came out I could see Glenn talking to this chap who had his back to me but was dressed like a zookeeper. It wasn't until I got up to them that I could see he was holding this dear little baby wombat whose mother had been killed on the road. The baby was so cute I wanted to take it home with me. Glenn bought me a stuffed one instead, which I now use as a doorstop.

As I'd been staying with Glenn during the off-season, I still didn't realise just how well known he was. It wasn't until he and I were invited to a barbecue one evening by a couple who have since become good friends of ours, Bev and Darren Mitchell, that it finally dawned on me. We'd arrived at their flat and I'd been introduced to quite a few people and was mingling, as you do, when Bev, who's also English, casually dropped into our conversation, 'so what's it like going out with Glenn McGrath?' I was a little confused by the question and asked her what she meant, to which she replied, 'You know, with him being a superstar.' I was slightly taken aback, to say the least, and told her I didn't know what she was talking about. 'You mean like Ryan Giggs (a Manchester United football player)?' I asked, and she replied 'Who's he?' 'Exactly,' I said. 'He's a great football player but you haven't heard of him.' Her response to that was 'But Jane, Glenn's as famous as Robert De Niro.' My jaw almost hit the floor. I wasn't 100 per cent sure that she wasn't pulling my leg, so I decided to take Glenn to one side and have a word with him about all this, as I was now beginning to feel a bit of a fool. I'd just assumed, as we'd walked through Cronulla and along the beach and esplanade, that he was simply a popular bloke and knew a lot of people. There were always people shouting 'Glenn, mate', and 'ooh aah', though I wasn't quite sure what the ooh aah was all about. He played the whole thing down, though I know he secretly loved the Robert De Niro comparison—I was sorry I'd mentioned that bit! That's one of the great things about Glenn, he is so modest and down to earth that if you didn't know him, he'd never tell you he was one of the world's best fast bowlers, if not the best. It's just one of the many things I love about him.

I knew that leaving Glenn this time was going to be terribly difficult, and I was absolutely dreading the day I had to fly home. I'd stayed with him in Cronulla for two months and had the most fantastic time. As is often the case when you're having a great time, leaving day came all too quickly. I didn't want to go. I knew I'd fallen in love with him but couldn't bring myself to tell him. I'd come close a couple of times but chickened out at the last minute. Something kept stopping me—I guess it just didn't feel right yet. On my last night in Australia, he took me out for dinner at a beachside seafood restaurant. We had a beautiful meal—well, it looked beautiful, but I felt too sick to eat much of it. I had a restless night's sleep; I didn't want the next morning to come. We drove to the airport the next day and as I was a bit early for my flight, we went and had a cup of tea before I disappeared through the departure gate. By now, I was practically fighting back my tears. I could hardly bear to look at Glenn I was so upset, and I remember him saying to me, 'Jane, this isn't the end, you know, it's just the beginning.'

G Not long after I returned to Sydney from the Hong Kong Sixes trip I received Jane's letter, and reading her words brought back the memories of the fun time we had shared. I certainly hadn't forgotten her. But our attempts to contact one another by telephone had been frustrated by her flight attendant schedule and my summer ritual of living out of a suitcase as a professional cricketer. I was happy to receive the letter and I was even happier to read that she had a chance to fly to Australia in early December. If I wanted, Jane said, she would visit me. Did I?! To be honest I had no pre-conceived ideas about our impending meeting; I was a single guy enjoying life, and as far as I was concerned that wasn't going to change in a hurry. I was living the bachelor's dream, and without going into too much detail, you can take it from me that there is no shortage of women wanting to 'meet' top class sportsmen—

especially cricketers. Some of the young single players treat that as part of the overall package. I'm the first to admit I was no angel in that regard and before I settled down with Jane I certainly enjoyed myself. However, cricket was always my main priority. I learned early in the piece that a bloke can lose his focus—and form—by becoming too involved in the temptations of the party scene. I guess it was because I had seen so much of that scene that I appreciated the fact that when I first met Jane she didn't know me as Glenn McGrath the cricketer; she knew me only as an Aussie bloke with his mates in a foreign pub, and she still liked me. It meant a lot, and when we became romantically involved I knew Jane liked me for who I was, not what I was.

Nevertheless, when I think back to Jane's arrival to Perth I can't help but cringe a bit. I didn't meet her at the airport, but that was not through rudeness. When her flight landed we had a team meeting at our base, the Hyatt. These are never taken lightly. In those team talks we run through our tactics and strategies and pinpoint our opponent's strengths and weaknesses. No one is excused from them. While Jane knew well in advance that I wouldn't be on hand to meet her, I feared my absence didn't send out much of a message to a lady who had travelled halfway across the planet to spend some time with me. At least I didn't have any official commitments that night, so I could at least devote the night to her.

So, after many missed phone calls and a valued letter, the girl I'd met in Hong Kong knocked on my door. It's funny, but when I saw Jane in the hallway—smiling nervously—I didn't feel the slightest hint of awkwardness; it was like greeting an old friend. Most of the boys had gone out for something to eat, but rather than trudge around Perth in search of a decent restaurant I ordered room service, and we talked for hours. We didn't miss a beat from where we left off in Hong Kong. However,

Jane did admit she'd had second thoughts about flying all the way to Australia for a fellow she hardly knew (I've always maintained the Narromine charm attracted her as sugar does a bee). My response was that we should not worry about things like that, but simply enjoy our time together. I guess that best reflects my attitude to life, which has always been to take everything as it comes.

Jane is a conscientious person, so before she winged her way Down Under she did some cricket homework; she bought a book of rules, and, like a student studying for an exam, crammed like crazy! She tried to understand what bowling a maiden over really meant, as well as coming to grips with other terms such as Leg Before Wicket, Wide, No Ball, Dead Ball, Night Watchman and Caught Behind. She wasn't the first to be confused by the many intricacies of the ancient game; I believe cricket is perhaps the hardest sport on earth to explain to someone not familiar with the rules. I guess the fact that even at 50 years of age Australia's greatest fast bowler, Dennis Lillee, said he too was still learning new things about the game says plenty about its complexity.

Anyway, Jane had five days to put her newfound knowledge to the test—I gave her a pass to watch each and every day of the encounter against the Sri Lankans. I had no idea of where she'd be sitting and couldn't find her among the sea of faces visible from my fielding position in the outfield at the WACA. I knew she was there, though. When I'm out on the paddock I focus fully on the cricket, but that day I sometimes found myself hoping Jane was all right by herself—I'm well aware that eight hours of cricket can be pretty tedious for someone who doesn't have a feel for it. I love the game with a passion, but even I struggle watching it from the outer—I'm one of those people who much prefers playing to watching from the stands. As for Jane being happy, I need not have worried. As I quickly learned, one of Jane's great attributes is that she can entertain herself. Like me she's content with her own company, and in between watching the Aussies wrestle with the Sri Lankans, she read a book in the sunshine and relaxed. However, I was taken aback later at the hotel when I asked for her thoughts on the day's play. Jane was pleased I took a few wickets, but the main memory she had of her First Class 'debut' was a desire to tear all her clothes off and run naked around the field! She said the sun and the sight of the soft green grass got to her. I didn't say a word, but I kept grinning . . .

The day after the Test I got to show Jane around Cronulla. It is a beautiful area, alive with birdlife, blessed with beautiful walks and far enough away from the city to get away from it all. The Sutherland Shire is very important to me, and I surprised even myself a few years ago when I told someone I intended to drop anchor in the area when I retire. When I left Narromine, at breakneck pace and in a cloud of dust, I figured I would one day return to the bush but now, after what feels like a lifetime by the surf and bush of the Royal National Park, I'm not so sure.

It didn't take much coaxing for my love of Cronulla to rub off on Jane. Like me, she's very much into nature—I'm told that when she was a child she only needed to see a rabbit hop across the lawn or a squirrel run along the back fence to make her happy for the rest of the day. The simple things in life please her most of all, and in those first few days in Australia she developed a fascination with kookaburras. Maybe it's because, like her, they like to laugh at all hours of the day. However, she was saddened to hear the male commits suicide by diving head-first into the ground when its mate dies . . . the loss is so bad for the bird his life isn't worth living. I might have made a joke of it then, but in time I was to learn that love—real love—for someone can supersede everything else. Jane appreciated the beauty of Mother Nature a lot more than many Aussies and quickly fell in love with the open spaces of Australia.

But still, Jane's week in the Great South Land quickly came to an end and she reluctantly packed her bags to return to the bite of the northern hemisphere's winter. I felt a great sorrow in seeing her go because during our time together Jane had confirmed everything I thought of her that first night in Hong Kong. She was warm, rich in humour, and caring, and her inner beauty was as obvious as her physical beauty. We again promised to keep in touch, and within days of her departure the pair of us were racking up expensive phone bills to say hello and keep tabs on each other's life.

Through our correspondence and numerous phone calls following her trip I could tell Jane was someone special, a woman of depth and substance. I looked forward to our marathon telephone conversations, even though they were at all hours of the night because of the time difference between the two hemispheres. It didn't take too long for me to identify Jane's distinctive handwriting, and I looked forward to seeing my latest letter from her when I made one of my rare trips to clear my post office box. There was obviously a bond growing between us—at a spectacular rate of knots—but it was hard to foster a relationship when we were separated by 20,000 kilometres, and our careers.

Jane's first visit in Perth came on the heels of an exhausting schedule. The Australian team had played gruelling Tests and one dayers in just about every corner of cricket's far-flung empire, and it took plenty out of us individually and as a squad. We players needed time to catch our breath and rest our muscles and minds. To their credit, the Cricket Board's hierarchy realised we needed time off, and allocated a four-to-five month break for us. It was not only a welcome respite from tour life but it also presented a perfect opportunity for me to invite Jane out to spend more time with me in Australia.

I planned for us to sit under a swaying palm tree in tropical North Queensland and sip cocktails while the world passed us by. I figured that would be the perfect place for Jane and me to get to know one another without the distractions and demands of our professional lives.

This time I was there—and on time (though Jane disagrees)—when she touched down in Australia. We just picked up from where we left off. I couldn't have been happier, and nor, I believe, could Jane. She is such a vivacious person that I sometimes see the world through her eyes, and it really is bright, big and beautiful. When it comes to sharing her emotions Jane is very uninhibited, and I'm happy to say it was plain for everyone in the arrival lounge to see that she was as glad to see me as I was to see her. But she had hardly any time to let her feet touch the ground because we weren't in Sydney for too long. I had been advised that Bloomfield was the slice of paradise I hankered for. One feature which really appealed to me was the fact it was secluded and private . . . there are never more than ten or twelve couples on the island at a time. The many trials and tribulations of the cricket field were left behind us, and while Jane may have been an experienced air hostess and witnessed some amazing sights during her working life I felt that the view spread out beneath our chartered flight from Cairns was one she'd long remember. I will.

The resort is set amid dense rainforests—it was like staying in the Garden of Eden, with the squawking cockatoos, screeching lorikeets and ever-present sweet scent of bougainvillea. And, just like Adam and Eve, Jane and I went on long, romantic walks through the forest and even danced in the moonlight. I was happy about a lot of things during that trip, but what made me happiest was Jane. She was beautiful, caring and extremely good company... I'd never known a person who could smile at just about anything.

However, there was some trouble in paradise and the trouble was my own, stupid fault. I put my foot in my big mouth when a fellow holidaymaker asked whether Jane and I were an 'item': without thinking, I said we were just friends. Good friends, but just friends. Well, didn't I see the storm set in her eyes! The look I received was icy, to say the least. In hindsight, I probably deserved it. In my defence, all I can say is that while Jane is now my best friend, back then, we were simply friends. But still I should have been more sensitive to Jane's feelings.

Luckily the tropical sun soon thawed the frost and we participated in a number of the resort's activities together. I even managed to fulfil a long-held dream when I tried scuba diving, with Jane by my side 10 deep metres under the waves, on the floor of the Coral Sea. It was an amazing experience. My first reaction was to panic — it takes some time to relax after you take the initial plunge. It's hard to breathe normally, and the only noise I could hear was the gasping, raspy sound of my own breath... it was like being in the movie *Alien*. I could tell Jane felt the same, because her eyes were as big as saucers! But even though she was frightened, she didn't budge an inch; she stayed with me until the bitter end.

We returned to the city suntanned and in one piece. When we did the rounds it pleased me no end to realise that my friends recognised the same qualities I admired about Jane. I wasn't after the mob's vote of approval, but I was happy she was a hit all the same. During Jane's stay we went to a couple of weddings including that of my New South Wales team-mate Neil Maxwell. Neil tied the knot at Taronga Zoo, on the foreshores of sparkling Sydney Harbour, and it was magic.

Personally, I would have picked a lion or a snow leopard, but in their wisdom the newly married Mr and Mrs Maxwell decided upon a cute 'n cuddly little wombat and Jane loved him. I think her reaction—unbridled squeals of delight—stole the wombat's thunder.

Our time together gave Jane a false impression about my lifestyle. She was still trying to get her head around the concept of me being a professional cricketer, and I think she thought my life was just a matter of playing a few games in summer and spending months at home in the winter. She couldn't have been further off the mark. I explained that I was sometimes on the road for up to eight months at a time. Few international cricket teams are in the kind of demand the Australian outfit is, and more often than not, our winters are spent trudging through Sri Lanka, Zimbabwe, South Africa and Bangladesh. I had to put her in the picture—and fast: I didn't want her to think I had too easy a time!

LOVE HURTS

J Going back to my life in England was so hard. Glenn was on my mind the whole time—I just couldn't get him out of my head. We talked on the telephone at least once a week but it simply wasn't enough any more. I couldn't see how the situation was ever going to be any different. We talked about meeting up in Hong Kong. When the boys were away on tour, they usually stopped off in Hong Kong as the team was then sponsored by Cathay Pacific, a Hong Kong-based airline. They generally toured overseas about twice a year, so this prospect didn't exactly fill me with too much excitement. It just wasn't enough. My life was revolving around getting my monthly roster and then trying to shuffle my flights so that I'd have enough time off to fly out to Sydney and see him. Virgin had excellent staff concessions, and with my long service, it meant I could fly out from London to Sydney via Hong Kong for around $300, which was nothing.

But I couldn't think about anything else and it was doing my head in. I was putting myself under enormous pressure and it seemed to be getting me nowhere. Now I knew I loved him. I still hadn't told him, which just added to my frustrations. It was during one of our long telephone conversations that Glenn finally told me he loved me (Glenn remembers this differently!). I was so relieved to be able to tell him at last how I felt. It was as though a huge weight had been lifted from me, and the fact that he felt the same was just brilliant. But it still didn't change anything. I still lived in a sleepy little village in the Cotswolds and he lived on the other side of the world, in Sydney. I also knew that although he loved me, his cricketing career was taking off and that still had to come first. The last thing he needed in his life was a girlfriend who was going to put pressure on him, and I was determined never to become that.

With the help of a friend in Virgin who knew of my situation, I was finally able to rearrange my flights so that I still did the same number of flights in a month but also managed to get a full week off in between—and I planned another visit. I decided that, for my sanity's sake, this would have to be my last trip to Sydney. I would have to tell Glenn that the distance was just too great and being apart from him was breaking my heart. My life had become consumed with finding ways to be with him and it was tearing me apart. The bottom line was I simply couldn't do this to myself any longer.

When I landed in Sydney and saw him again waiting for me in the Arrivals hall, my heart was pounding. It was so great to see him again, but it simply reaffirmed my belief that this situation could not continue. For my own self-preservation, I told him the day after I arrived that I wouldn't be flying to Sydney again. I think he was a little shocked, but he understood how I felt. After all, I was the one doing all the trans-continental to-ing and fro-ing whilst he concentrated on his cricket. Glenn's response was for me to wait and see how I felt by the end of the week and make my decision then. But my mind was already made up.

We had a wonderful week together, just relaxing and enjoying each other's company. On the Friday evening (I was leaving that weekend), we were invited out to dinner at the yacht club by Bev and Darren. We were having a really lovely evening when, out of the blue, Glenn took me to one side and asked me if I'd leave England and live with him in Cronulla. I could not believe my ears. After thinking about it for roughly ten seconds, I said that yes, I'd be prepared to give it a go. There were no promises of an engagement, no guarantees. We just agreed to see how we went and take it one step at a time. I'd been taking chances in our relationship ever since I'd first known him, so this was really no different. To me, it was definitely a risk worth taking, and in many respects, deciding to move out to Australia was one of the easiest decisions I've ever had to make. It just felt so right. After all, if the worst came to the worst and things didn't work out, I'd simply fly back to England and start again. I had nothing to lose and everything to gain. One thing was certain: I knew how much I loved him and that he was worth the gamble. I flew home, resigned from Virgin—after seven happy years—and put my little cottage up for rent.

G As our relationship had blossomed the tyranny of distance had become too much of a strain on Jane. It seemed we were forever dreaming up plans which could have been straight out of a James Bond novel; meeting in Hong Kong or Bangkok at 1500 hours for a weekend rendezvous, for instance. We plotted a number of similar crazy—and just as impractical—schemes; they were devised in a terrible desperation to spend more time together. Our relationship had fallen into a pattern of sorts, and while it was tremendous to feel so close to someone, it was also frustrating. We compensated for not being together with hastily scrawled post cards, deep and meaningful letters and very late night phone calls, and we tried to learn to live with that awful feeling of emptiness lovers feel when they're separated. Through her job with the airline Jane could get to Australia cheaply so it was she who battled the long, energy-draining flights and the onslaught of jet lag which would throw her system out of kilter for a few days at a time.

When she did come back for that one week stay it was as if we were trying to absorb as much energy as we could from one another to survive the next long break. The terrible drought. Jane then told me she wouldn't be back; the emotional drain of leaving was all too much for her. I think she knew how she felt about me for quite a while but she kept a lid on it. She had told me she loved me over the telephone on her return to the United Kingdom (of course Jane remembers this differently!), but I guess my nonchalant attitude towards being tied down gave her a good reason to keep check on her feelings. Indeed, she was a bit like me when I was a young bloke and I didn't dare tell anyone why I bowled at that 44-gallon drum for hours at a time—I feared being ridiculed and, worse still, rejected.

While I knew from the start that Jane was special, I fought her attempts to cement our relationship. After all, I was young, single and living the life of Riley. I was happy in myself and was in no rush to change things . . . at least not until the day before Jane was ready to return to England—for good this time. We were at the Port Hacking Game Fishing Club and it wasn't the happiest of occasions. Jane was gearing up to return home and our best efforts to be cheerful were defeated by the dread of yet another awful farewell at the airport—the low point was always the abrupt feeling of emptiness that overwhelmed us when Jane went through the doors leading into Customs. Right there at the restaurant table I realised the truth—I didn't want her to leave me. When she said it would be her last trip, it was like hearing a bell ring . . . in an instant the world as I knew it crumbled into a heap. The facade I'd built around me proved very flimsy indeed. I asked her to move to Australia.

I had already searched my heart about Jane earlier that day when I was out fishing on Port Hacking. Sometimes I think a person can find a lot of answers to life's questions when they're at one with nature; it's amazing how clear a bloke's head can get when he's out on the water or in the bush. I had thought long and hard about Jane leaving for England, and somewhere in between hooking a bream and returning to shore I had subconsciously prepared myself to ask her to leave Britain. When I sat at that table and heard her open her heart I was overwhelmed by a feeling of complete and utter devotion. Within seconds I asked her to take the big plunge and kiss England goodbye.

She said yes straight away, despite it being a huge decision. Her father wasn't so sure. Roy is a conservative gent, and I guess the idea of Jane packing up to be with a fast bowler on the other side of the world didn't rest easy with him as he watched Jane toss in a great job, get rid of her belongings and rent out her house in the Cotswolds all on a seeming whim.

When Jane had told me she couldn't bear the pain of being apart it struck a chord within me—I couldn't bear the thought that the next time I farewelled her at the airport could be the last time I'd see her either. Up until that point I'd had the upper hand in the relationship: I had my cricket, I was a bloke—and an Aussie bloke at that—and my life was free and easy. However, in a second I surrendered everything, and I did so freely. My life before meeting Jane was pretty good, but I can assure you it's been a lot bloody better with her, despite one or two hurdles fate placed in our paths.

LOVE HURTS

But Jane was given a harsh initiation into the realities of being a Test cricketer's partner. After severing all her ties to fly Down Under, her landing was anything but soft. I was away on tour when she arrived and there was no one to greet her. Rather than being overwhelmed by kisses and a bouquet of flowers, she was left to go to Cronulla alone and wait for another campaign to end.

Part Two

OUR NEW LIFE

A FEARFUL DISCOVERY

On 4 September 1996, I drove down to Heathrow airport to catch my flight to a new life in Australia. My Dad met me at the airport. He wanted to say goodbye, and there were a few things regarding my cottage that I needed to leave with him. We had a cup of tea and a chat and soon it was time for me to go. I was so excited, but I must admit to having a tear in my eye as I went through the departure gate. I think Dad did too. Well, there was no going back now. At this stage, it all felt rather like a dream, as if it wasn't really happening. I attempted to calm my nerves with a glass of champagne and tried to get some sleep but I was too excited. Twelve hours later, we landed in Hong Kong and I caught my flight to Sydney. I was over halfway there and it still didn't feel real. Finally we touched down in Sydney. I'd arrived. Unfortunately, Glenn was away playing in the Singer World Series in Sri Lanka, and wouldn't be home for another couple of days, so I collected my luggage (just the two suitcases) and caught a taxi to his flat in Cronulla. It was another perfect day, not a cloud in the sky. I walked into my new home, dropped my bags and fell onto the bed. I was absolutely exhausted but had never been happier.

Glenn arrived home from the Sri Lankan tour three days later and I drove to the airport to meet him. When I got to the Arrivals hall, I spotted a group of glamorous blonde girls (hard to miss!) who I thought must be the other players' wives and girlfriends. I'd gone along in my jeans and a t-shirt so I just stood on the other side of the hall right at the back, hiding. It was then that I noticed all the television cameras and wondered who would be coming through; maybe someone famous was in town. I nearly died when, a few minutes later, the cricket team came walking through in their stripy blazers and the flashes started going off and the cameras began rolling—the media were waiting for them! Then I saw Glenn come through. You can't really miss him in that blazer! I watched him scanning the crowds. He didn't see me at first, hiding in the furthest corner, but then he spotted me and beckoned me over. I was mortified at the prospect of having to walk over to him in front of all those people and felt rooted to the spot. He called me again and I reluctantly began to walk over to him. He gave me a big hug and a kiss and said he'd like to introduce me to the other players and girls. I would have preferred to run away but he insisted. We walked over to the other girls and their partners. Stephen's wife, Lynette, had brought their new baby girl, Rosalie, to the airport, and everyone was very excited to see them. Glenn introduced me but no one seemed to take much notice. I wanted to leave immediately. They probably thought I was just his latest fling. That was my first real taste of public life with Glenn and it had come as a bit of a shock.

Three weeks later, the team was off again. It was to India this time and once again, I found myself back at the airport

A FEARFUL DISCOVERY

with him, this time saying goodbye. I dropped Glenn off at Departures with all his luggage and drove off to park the car. He'd told me to meet him back at the Cathay check-in desk. As I walked towards the desk, I could see Glenn, along with a couple of the other boys, still waiting in line to check in their bags. I stood to the side at a distance, feeling very awkward and not really sure where to put myself. It was then that I noticed a couple of the other girls standing close to the check-in desk. One of them waved to me and called me over. It was a small gesture but I was so grateful for it. I walked over and Susan Porter, Mark Waugh's fiancée, introduced herself and her daughter Lauren to me. Enter Tracy Bevan. Glenn had told me about Tracy, how she was also English and the same age as me and I'd at first had high hopes for our friendship. We seemed to have so much in common. Unfortunately for me, these hopes were quickly quashed when Glenn then informed me that he'd previously been out with a good friend of Tracy's and finished with her for me. So Tracy might not be too keen to get to know me at all. Susan introduced us and sure enough, she didn't seem too interested in me. Thankfully, the boys appeared and we went off to grab a quick bite to eat before it was time for them to go. Then we walked to the departure gate, where the Slaters and Stephen and Lynette were saying their goodbyes, all tearful. I gave Glenn a kiss and a hug goodbye and he was gone. The other girls were a mess, telling me the goodbyes get more and more difficult as time goes on. 'Great,' I thought. When the boys had gone, we were all left feeling a bit flat. Tracy suggested we go for a coffee and a chat, to which everyone readily agreed. Although I was keen to join them, I'd left my purse in the car and didn't have any cash on me. I'd only just met them and didn't feel exactly close enough just yet to ask them to shout me a cappuccino, so I hesitated. Tracy took this as me being standoffish, and so I had to confess to her that I was rather embarrassed as I didn't have any cash on me. They shouted me my coffee and we haven't looked back since.

With Glenn away so often I decided I needed a cat for company. I've always had a great love for animals, particularly our feline friends—growing up, we always had a cat. Glenn wasn't keen at all, as he'd never been particularly fond of them. Being brought up on a farm, he considered them more of a pest than a pet. He eventually relented and agreed, but it had to be a Siamese. That was fine by me. I was lucky enough to find a breeder of pedigree cats right there in Cronulla, not far from where we lived. She had some beautiful cats, and many different breeds, but we fell in love with Simba, a chocolate point Siamese who I'm sure thinks he's a dog most of the time! One of his favourite toys is an old purple bikini top of mine which he took a liking to whilst Glenn and I were overseas in England on the '97 Ashes tour. He drags it around in his mouth like a security blanket, and likes you to throw it for him so that he can bring it back to you. A few months after getting Simba, Glenn agreed to us getting another cat as company for Simba, this time for the occasions when Glenn and I both went away! I returned to the local breeder looking for another Siamese. She told me she had a black Oriental who had been one of a pair. His brother had been sold and the buyer hadn't wanted two cats so the other little fella had been left alone. I wasn't really that interested as I thought Orientals were all ears and legs, but after hearing that story I agreed to have a look. He was actually very cute, a real character, and when I picked him up and gave him a cuddle he purred like a motorbike! I immediately fell in love with him and took him home. We named him Tigger because he was just a bundle of energy and bounced around all over the place. Poor Simba didn't get a moment's peace from that day on. They were great company and I absolutely adored them.

As the months passed and things were working out really well between us, Glenn and I decided it was time for me to apply for my residency. Anyone that's had to do this will know what a long process it is and that part of that process involves you constantly having to prove to the Department of Immigration that your relationship is genuine and ongoing. Apart from bills and Christmas cards, I was in the unusual position of being able to send them newspaper clippings about us—articles saying how much in love we were. Still, I didn't expect any preferential treatment because of the high-profile nature of our relationship, and we didn't get any. I was absolutely thrilled when I was eventually granted my residency two years later, in March 1999.

In May 1997, I flew back to England with a few of the other wives and girlfriends for the Ashes tour. It was good to see England again—not that I'd missed it—especially the familiar sights like Marks & Spencer. The best thing was seeing my family and friends, of course. The girls were not allowed to stay with the boys for the first six weeks of the tour (so that some good old male bonding could go on), so during that time I stayed with Mum at her home in Lichfield, Staffordshire, and visited other friends. On one occasion, the team was staying at a beautiful country club called Breadsall Priory, which was near Derby and not too far from Mum's. As she and Glenn hadn't met yet it seemed like a good opportunity, so my mum, Jen, invited Glenn around for dinner. She cooked roast chicken, enough for an army, and we all enjoyed a very relaxed evening.

The First Test on tour was at Edgbaston, Birmingham, and Australia had the biggest shock when they were beaten by England. I think the England team was probably just as shocked. After the match, Tracy and I went down to the players' bar to wait for Michael and Glenn, knowing that our men would be absolutely stunned, as we were. A few of the England players were down in the bar, and Darren Gough was one of them. Michael used to play county cricket for Yorkshire, Darren's club, so Tracy took me over to say hello and introduce me. We begrudgingly congratulated him on England's win and I couldn't resist following my congratulations up with, 'Make the most of it, it won't last long'.

I really enjoyed the Ashes tour, not only for the cricket but also for the socialising. The boys got to play golf at St Andrews and the Belfry and went for a drive around the Grand Prix racetrack, and since we were in England during June, anyone interested was invited to go to Wimbledon for the lawn tennis and, of course, the most delicious strawberries and cream. We also went to the theatre in London to see *Les Misérables*. At the end of the tour, the whole team and their partners went on an evening cruise down the river Thames that was put on by Coca-Cola, the Australian team tour sponsors. We had a great night gently cruising along the Thames, under Tower Bridge, past Big Ben and the Houses of Parliament, St Paul's Cathedral and all the way down to the Thames Barrier. There was a live band playing on board, but they were later ousted by an impromptu performance by Shane Lee and Michael Slater with Michael Bevan on lead vocals. A night to remember—or maybe to quickly forget!

In between the Test matches, the boys played against the various English counties. It was now August and the game

A FEARFUL DISCOVERY

before the final Test at The Oval was against Kent, down in Canterbury. Canterbury is an extremely old and beautiful town in the south of England. Many of the buildings in the main street, which is now a pedestrian mall, are Tudor, with black and white exteriors, and wooden beams and low ceilings on the inside. The stunning cathedral is also on the main street in the centre of town. We were lucky enough to be staying at a hotel on the main street that was convenient for the cricket ground, for shopping and for eating out in the evening. It was during our brief stay in Canterbury that I first discovered the lump in my left breast. I had just taken my morning shower and was standing in front of the bathroom mirror with a towel around my waist, combing my wet hair through. As I stood and combed my hair, my gaze was continually drawn to a section of my left breast and I became convinced that, somehow, it didn't look right. I told myself not to be silly, and began putting on my make-up, but still the feeling wouldn't go away. Alarm bells started to sound in my head. Mum had been diagnosed with breast cancer when she was forty-nine, and had had to have a mastectomy. I had felt for her so much and admired her courage in beating this life-threatening illness. In spite of the fact that this had happened to her, I never in a million years dreamt that it might happen to me too. There are so many possible causes of breast cancer. Research to date shows that less than five per cent of all breast cancer is hereditary. I knew Mum had been under a lot of stress and I was sure this was the reason behind her illness. I'd see articles in *Elle* and *Cosmo* about breast cancer and always skim past them. Looking back now, I don't know how or why I was so sure I'd be immune to the disease, but I was. Not one of Mum's doctors or medical team had approached me following her illness, and I guess I felt that if they weren't concerned about how her breast cancer could affect me, then I didn't have to worry. I've since learnt that you have to be responsible for your own wellbeing and look after yourself. If you don't care about yourself and your health, how can you expect anyone else to?

I examined my breast, and I couldn't actually feel a lump. But the feeling that something was terribly wrong became overwhelming. The breast just didn't look right. Instead of being curved underneath, it appeared to flatten out on one side. In the end, I felt my breast so much that I made it sore, which convinced me that I couldn't possibly have cancer as I'd been told that cancerous lumps aren't painful. I was clutching at straws, of course; I know that now. Glenn was lying on the bed watching television and so I went out to him and asked him if he could feel a lump or if my breast looked strange to him. He couldn't see anything wrong but he could see that I was upset and suggested that we go and visit my doctor up in the Cotswolds, just to put my mind at ease. I said no, it was probably nothing, just my imagination running riot, although deep down I knew something was very wrong, and the voice in my head kept on telling me the same. The Bevans were in the room opposite ours and I rearranged my towel and nipped across the hallway to see Tracy. I told her how I was feeling, but didn't show her the breast, and in about ten minutes I had managed to talk myself out of the whole thing. I went back to our room, got dressed and tried to forget all about it.

Australia went on to win the 1997 Ashes series, and on Thursday, 28 August, we all left for Sydney, expecting to arrive home on Saturday, 30 August. Due to the conditions of my bridging visa (my residency still not having been granted at this stage), I had to be back in Sydney no later than 31 August 1997. A couple of the boys knew about this. Glenn

A FEARFUL DISCOVERY

and I were lucky enough to be sitting in front of Mark Taylor on the flight home. Just after I'd woken up from a couple of hours' sleep I was informed by him whispering in my ear that our plane had developed a technical problem and we were having to divert, which meant we'd be a day late into Sydney. I nearly had a heart attack and had visions of being refused entry into Australia and sent straight back to London. He thinks he's funny, does Mark. He'll keep!

We'd been back at home in Cronulla for a couple of days when we were invited round for dinner with our friends, Bev and Darren. It was Wednesday, 3 September. We hadn't seen them since before the Ashes tour, and had lots of catching up to do. We were both looking forward to the evening. While we'd been overseas, Bev had decided to have her breasts reduced. The operation had been a great success and she asked me if I'd like to see them, which of course I did. They looked great and she was really pleased with them. As we chatted away on the subject of breasts, I decided to take the opportunity to ask her about mine, particularly as Bev is a theatre sister. I took a deep breath and told her that I felt there was something wrong with my left breast and at the same time tried to make light of it. She offered to have a look at it for me and I reluctantly agreed. Reluctantly, because I realised that this was finally going to be the moment of truth. She told me to lie down on the bed, which surprised me as I'd been examining my breast standing up. She explained that it was sometimes easier to feel a lump when you're lying down, as the breast spreads out more. Anyway, I took off my top and lay down on her bed. She examined my breast and said that, yes, she could definitely feel a lump there. My heart sank. She had confirmed what I had known inside since that morning in Canterbury two weeks earlier, and now I could no longer ignore it. My eyes began to fill with tears but I fought them back, got dressed and we walked back into the lounge, where the boys were talking over a beer. I beckoned to Glenn and told him Bev had said that she could feel a lump there. He went to hug me but I told him not to—I knew I'd crumble if he did and I wanted us to stay and have dinner and a good evening as we'd planned. I didn't have my own doctor at this point and Bev offered to call her doctor, explain my situation and make an appointment for me for first thing the next morning.

G Every Australian cricketer's dream is to tour the cradle of cricket—England—on an Ashes campaign, so even though it was expected, it was still an almighty thrill for me to hear my name read out as part of Mark Taylor's 17-man squad for the 106-day 1997 tour. I'm sure I can speak on behalf of the other blokes when I say we felt the full weight of the nation's expectation on our shoulders as we packed our kit bags.

Some critics thought the English selectors had picked a team of players capable of teaching us a lesson and they were quick to point this out after the home team's victory in the First Test at Birmingham. I had onfield problems with my line and length on the English pitches; the problems began with my run-up. I just didn't feel right, and the Englishmen made the most of my frustrations by hitting a total of 149 runs off my bowling for the loss of just two wickets. However, with extra training—which included returning to Edgbaston the day after the Test loss to bowl at one stump—things fell back into place.

Despite the harsh initiation I rate being outfitted with my official Ashes blazer a crowning moment in my career. It was the realisation of a childhood dream; the memory of being banished to the outfield for the Backwater XI because of a supposed lack of ability seemed a lifetime away. While that tour was to provide me with one of my career highlights—the eight wicket haul in the first innings of the Lord's Test—it would also see Jane's and my life sent into a terrible spin.

Our romance had blossomed and the love we shared was growing deeper every day. There were few, if any, problems and because we had so much in common I figured I'd found my soulmate. I wanted Jane's stay in Australia to be a more permanent one, but the amount of red tape we had to hack through was mind-boggling—and bloody frustrating. While I made numerous calls and petitioned anyone I thought could help, I honestly had no idea if her application would be rubber-stamped. The feeling of trepidation frustrated me no end, because Jane Steele wasn't just another statistic or a 'candidate for immigration' . . . she was the person I was banking on growing old with; the person I planned to share my innermost thoughts and dreams with. My best attempts to explain such thoughts seemed to go straight over the heads of the public servants. In hindsight—and in their defence—I can imagine they're bombarded with similar stories on a daily basis.

It had never crossed my mind that Jane might be rejected and when that thought hit home I couldn't help but feel edgy. Not just for our relationship's sake, but also because Jane had given up her cottage and sold her belongings to start a new life with me. Also, for a bloke who prides himself on being in control of his life, I was dirty on myself for not anticipating any potential problems . . . and this was one heck of a problem. We at least had a sanctuary to escape our hassles: a 13,770-hectare property situated 100 kilometres beyond the back of Bourke. The boundary fence almost touches the Queensland border. The Cuttaburra River runs through the property, which is home to an assortment of native animals, including colonies of kangaroos and emus. Jane thought of the place as a little piece of heaven until the time it was invaded by a couple of mice; for some reason she doesn't appear to be so keen on going bush now. I find the place is good for my soul, and I look forward to the day I finally gain my helicopter pilot's licence—being able to lift off from Hoxton Park airport about forty kilometres from home will spare me a ten-hour car trip. I'm sure even Jane will agree nothing is as conducive to thinking about the big picture as sitting on the front verandah of our homestead and toasting yet another glorious sunset with a nice, icy cold drink.

Given the hassles, I was pleasantly surprised when the Department of Immigration gave Jane permission to leave the country and accompany me on part of the Ashes tour while her residency application was being processed. Jane, who would follow about a month later, saw me off at Sydney's International Airport, but it was hard to show too much emotion—the departure terminal was crammed with photographers, television cameras, journalists, autograph hunters and other well-wishers. I find I'm very self-conscious in such a situation and when I think of the 'fish-bowl' it's little wonder my good mate Steve Waugh usually says his goodbyes to his wife Lynette at their home because he finds the kind of distractions Jane and I encountered an unwelcome imposition.

While Australians have long enjoyed 'hating' the Poms I must admit I liked England. The history of the place—and the people—really appealed to me. Most of the Brits I met were tremendous, but there was a small group of 'fans' who went to

A FEARFUL DISCOVERY

the cricket with what seemed to be the express purpose of giving me a hard time, and I admit there were times I wished a few of Narromine's hardest nuts were in the outer to sort them out. They made abusive comments ranging from we Aussies supposedly being born out of wedlock to being of convict stock. The yobbos were the exception rather than the rule and most of the people I met in England, Jane's friends especially, were very hospitable. England is steeped in history and you can't help but feel it everywhere you go. I especially enjoyed visiting the major tourist attractions, such as the Tower of London and Buckingham Palace, where the team was presented to the Queen and Prince Andrew. That was the occasion when my fast bowling buddy Michael Kasprowicz tried to entice Her Majesty to show the fellows a few moves straight from the 'Gladiators' at the Military Tattoo.

After a disappointing effort in the opening Test we steadied the ship and when we fired our next broadside at the English XI they had no idea what hit them. Mark Taylor ended a rut when he scored a century; Jason Gillespie emerged as a world-class fast bowler; Steve Waugh put the Brits to his sword with murderous results; and I bagged a few wickets, including a career best, 8-38, at the home of cricket, Lord's. It is a tremendous source of pride for me to think that the name and figures G.D. McGrath 8-38 are written on an honour board in the visitors' dressing room alongside such greats as Keith Miller and Bob Massie. The board commemorates every batsman who scores a century or any bowler who has bagged five wickets in an innings there and straight after we skittled the Pommies for a lousy 77 it floored me when I saw the then Australian coach Geoff Marsh had beaten the ground's signwriter to his job by scribbling my name on some white tape and putting it on the board. It's things like the honour board which make Lord's so special. What stands out most in my mind when I think of the home of cricket is the silence of the place as I ran in to bowl the first fast ball of our war. In every other Test ground around the world, an almighty din accompanies every step of the opening bowler's run in. But not at Lord's . . . I've never experienced anything like it, and it helps make the memory of my best bowling effort in Test cricket even more special.

Jane and my mother were in the crowd, and having them there added to the occasion. Indeed, Jane earned the wrath of the attendants in the stuffy Members area when she was told to sit down and be quiet—she was screaming her lungs out as I walked off the field with the rest of the boys. And I reckon they would have reached boiling point when they realised she was an English lass cheering on an Aussie! That Ashes series was different from many of the other tours we had embarked upon because most of the players' partners made the trip. As the two 'locals' of the group, Jane and Tracy Bevan led the charge to the shops and other places of interest on the girls' outings. Actually, being in England provided me with a greater insight into Jane's life and her upbringing. I met her family; I saw where she went to school; I was given the tour of her grandmother's old sweet shop and I even saw the backyard pavers Jane enjoyed scrubbing as a kid! She thought it was great fun. We did the rounds of her relatives and drove down to her mother's place at Lichfield for dinner. While there are always nerves about meeting a girlfriend's family for the first time I don't think the meeting could have gone better; the meal was very relaxed and informal.

However, in Canterbury a dirty, dark cloud appeared on our trip to England together, and eventually it unleashed an emotional storm which left us reeling. I initially dismissed those fears of Jane as she stood combing her hair in front of the mirror as nothing to sweat over, because I figured at just thirty-one Jane was too young to suffer what is universally considered an older woman's disease. I didn't think she had anything to worry about and I told her so a million times. When I read a brochure on breast cancer it seemed my reason for not panicking was well justified: apparently 90 per cent of all lumps in women aged under forty are benign. So I figured she was being silly. Even though I could see the worry in Jane's eyes, I remained relaxed about it. Indeed, my devil-may-care attitude was mirrored by Tracy Bevan when Jane sought her counsel in their room across the hallway. After that 'second opinion' Jane made a conscious decision not to worry about it, but not knowing what was wrong with her tormented her. Now I can imagine what having to deal with the dark thoughts which pervaded her mind at night must have been like—sheer bloody hell. When I realised the worry of the lump was tearing Jane apart I advised her to see a doctor—no matter how bad the news, it would be better to know what was wrong. But Jane was terrified that if she did have breast cancer the doctor would not allow her to leave for Australia in time to beat the Immigration Department's deadline. I thought she was crazy, talking of cancer. At worst, I figured it might be a cyst. When we left England I was convinced it was nothing—you know, the old Aussie approach of 'she'll be apples mate'—and simply hoped she could relax and sleep for a few hours during the long flight to Sydney.

Not long after we returned, Jane and I had dinner with our friends Darren and Bev Mitchell at their place. It was meant to be a celebration; after all, I was named Australia's Player-of-the-tour. We'd wrapped up the Ashes and according to some commentators I had also established myself as cricket's leading fast bowler. It was golden stuff, but Jane's dark frame of mind took some of the gloss off the night, and off the sense of achievement. All the doomsday talk was getting to me, so as we drove to our friends' home I insisted that Jane ask Bev to take a look at the lump. Bev is a registered nurse so I thought —hoped, really—she would be able to put an end to the drama by telling Jane she was being silly to worry herself about nothing. Sadly, I couldn't have been more off the mark. After she looked at the breast Bev urged Jane to waste no time in seeing a doctor. Not surprisingly, the urgency in Bev's voice really frightened Jane, and after weeks of penting up her deepest and darkest fears she lost it—albeit momentarily. When I saw tears well in her eyes I attempted to comfort her with a hug, but she didn't want that. Instead she applied the renowned British stiff upper lip and ate her dinner. But it wasn't the Jane I knew. Her trademark laughter was missing; she was withdrawn and I could practically hear the demons dancing up a storm in her mind. It was obvious she was trying to come to grips with a worst case scenario—a positive breast cancer diagnosis. While it was plain to see Jane was terrified, I clung to my belief that there was nothing to worry about. It's almost sad to admit this, but my solace was to simply shrug my shoulders and think tragedies such as breast cancer happen to other people, not Jane and me. I again took comfort in thinking breast cancer was an older woman's disease and at thirty-one Jane was far from old.

J My appointment with the doctor was for 9.40 am the next day—Thursday, 4 September. Glenn had a training session. He offered to cancel but I told him to go and not to worry, I'd be fine. I caught a taxi to the surgery and went in to see the doctor. I removed my top and lay down on the bed in the surgery while he carefully examined my breast. He then told me he could feel not one lump, but two. He explained that the

A FEARFUL DISCOVERY

chances of them being malignant were very low, considering my age. I was thirty-one. He said that the lumps were probably fibroid adenomas, but given the fact that Mum had had breast cancer, he suggested I go for a mammogram (an x-ray of the breast) and an ultrasound and to drop the results in when I was passing next. I was so reassured by what he said that I skipped out of that surgery. As it was such a sunny, beautiful day, I decided to walk home. Looking back now, it's hard to imagine why I was so happy having just been told I had two lumps in my breast, but I just remember that I was. I so desperately wanted to believe that everything was going to be alright, that it was all a fuss about nothing.

That evening, I thought it was about time I called my parents and let them know what was happening. I hadn't wanted to worry them unnecessarily, but Glenn and I decided they ought to know. I don't actually remember much about the phone calls apart from the fact that I desperately tried to make light of the situation in a bid to make it easier for them to deal with, especially as they were on the other side of the world and could really do nothing to help. I told them about the lumps and the doctor's prognosis and that, as a precautionary measure, I was going off for a mammogram and ultrasound the next day. I reassured them both that it was most likely that the lumps were fibroid adenomas, but I'd get them checked out and call them with the results. After all, it was better to be safe than sorry.

I tried to make my appointment for my mammogram and ultrasound for that Thursday afternoon, as Glenn's younger brother, Dale, was getting married in Dubbo that weekend and I really wanted to go with Glenn to the wedding and to see the rest of his family. We'd planned to leave Sydney early on the Friday morning to allow ourselves plenty of time for the five-hour journey. Unfortunately, having both a mammogram and an ultrasound in the same appointment takes quite a long time, and the Imaging Centre couldn't fit me in until Friday morning, which meant Glenn and I had to delay our trip to Dubbo for a few hours.

On Friday, 5 September, I went off to the Imaging Centre. Glenn had a few things to do that morning so I told him to meet me there when he could. Before I could go in for my mammogram I had to fill out the obligatory forms, and it was only then that I realised I didn't have any private health insurance. At this point, however, money was the least of my worries. I walked upstairs and took a seat in the waiting room, thumbing through a magazine without seeing what was on its pages until my name was called. I was led into a small room by a lovely lady who did her best to put me at ease. She told me to take off my top (by now I had become somewhat expert at this), and stand next to a tall machine, which was rather like an x-ray machine. I had to stand close enough to the machine to be able to place my breast on a cold metal plate. Another metal plate then clamped down on top of the breast, squashing it in, and the mammogram was taken. Several mammograms were taken from various angles on both breasts. The metal plates were cold and the squashing made my breasts tender, but I would describe it as more uncomfortable than painful. From here I went straight into the room next door for my ultrasound. For this, I had to lie down on a bed and the nurse applied a small amount of a jelly-like substance to my chest and then ran what looked like a microphone over my breasts. The idea is that this produces sound waves that a computer then turns into images—which are displayed on a monitor. On my ultrasound, you could see the two lumps at seven o'clock and nine o'clock, but the operator told me not to be too concerned as they were probably fibroid adenomas, reiterating what my doctor had said. I was feeling somewhat reassured until the lady who had taken my mammograms came in and said that the doctor had requested that she take a couple more, as a few of them weren't very clear. I was not convinced I was being told the whole truth and the alarm bells started sounding once more. I suddenly became very frightened and my eyes began to fill with tears. Nevertheless, I returned to the mammogram room and had several more taken. When all the examinations had been completed, I put my clothes back on, still fighting back the tears, and walked back to the waiting room, where I saw Glenn waiting for me. I was so relieved to see him I couldn't let him go. I explained to him what had happened and that I needed to go outside for some fresh air. As we had an hour to kill while we waited for the results, we decided to pop over to Miranda shopping mall and grab a bite to eat. It was now lunchtime. All I could think about were my results—I have no idea where we sat or what we had. I told Glenn I wanted to take my results straight down to my GP and not waste a second.

When we returned to the Imaging Centre an hour later to collect them, the lady behind the desk handed me a large white envelope containing my mammograms, with a fluoro yellow Post-It note stuck on it which read 'Doctor: 3pm'. Now I knew that something was dreadfully wrong. Why would they have bothered making an appointment for me? My heart sank.

We walked out to our car in a state of shock. As Glenn drove down to the surgery I sat there in the front passenger seat, quiet as a mouse with the envelope on my lap. I was looking at my name and seeing the word 'Mammogram' but I could not believe that this could be happening to me. It had to be an awful nightmare. Surely I'd wake up any second. But it wasn't a nightmare. In fact it was about to become all too real. Glenn and I walked into the surgery together, hand in hand, and gave my doctor the envelope with the tell-tale luminous Post-It note. We both sat down while he examined its contents. The expression on his face said it all. He informed us that things did not look good. The mammogram and ultrasound both indicated that there was indeed a problem but they alone did not confirm whether I actually had cancer or not. I would need to undergo a needle biopsy and this would tell us whether the lumps were benign or malignant. He also instructed me to immediately stop taking the contraceptive Pill which I had been on for about twelve years. All the time, I felt as though this was happening to someone else. It was as if I was floating above myself and looking down, watching it all happen. The doctor asked when I could go for the needle biopsy and Glenn and I agreed that the sooner the better and made an appointment for Monday, 8 September, the next working day. We walked back out to the car park hand in hand, both in shock, and climbed into the car. My eyes were full of tears and I turned to Glenn and whispered 'I've got cancer, haven't I?' I knew it and he didn't have to say a word. We sat there holding on to one another, unable to quite believe that this could all be happening.

G The walk back to the car park was like being in a daze . . . the doctor's words were ringing in my ears, and like Jane, I had fat tears in my eyes. And when she looked at me and said 'I've got cancer, haven't I?' there was nothing I could do, or say, except to hold her tight and long.

We were scheduled for a trip to Narromine for my brother Dale's wedding, but Jane wasn't up to it. Not only was she emotionally drained, but she was still stressed to the max. I could understand her reluctance—the long and dusty drive

A FEARFUL DISCOVERY

knocked the wind out of her at the best of times. I instead made the trip on my own, and most of my thoughts were with her ... I just wanted the drama to end and for us to resume the carefree life we had cherished so much. On hearing the circumstances surrounding Jane's absence, my family's response was one of complete understanding. Initially they were surprised to see me lob up alone because I decided to wait until I arrived to tell them. The family had met Jane a few times and they loved her, and their only comment on her absence was to hope that her fears would amount to nothing. My family was well aware of the pain of breast cancer because at around about that time my grandmother was also fighting the wretched disease.

To be brutally honest, while I was upset that Jane was so worried that she sometimes felt physically ill, I couldn't bring myself to believe she had anything to fear. The reason for that is that my life has long centred around not getting bogged down by 'ifs' and 'buts'. My approach has been to act on any problems and try and take control of a situation, be it on the cricket field, in the workplace, on the farm, in the bush or in my personal life. If I was to really examine my state of mind back then I would guess I was lax about Jane's plight because up until then I'd been spared any tragedies. Apart from my parents' divorce, about the worst thing that had happened to me as a kid was being overlooked for a starring role in my junior cricket team. I had an invincibility shield around me ... but it proved to be an illusion, because in the end it failed to protect Jane.

J There was still Dale and Sandy's wedding that weekend and Glenn had to go—he was in the bridal party. There was absolutely no way on earth I felt I could travel out to Dubbo for the wedding and pretend that everything was fine when we'd just been told that there was a strong possibility I had breast cancer. I was a complete and utter mess. Glenn wanted to stay with me but he had no choice. He couldn't miss his brother's wedding and I insisted that he went. Life goes on. I was happy to spend the weekend at home alone. It would give me some time to pull myself together and get my head around the enormity of the events of the past week. Everything had happened so quickly.

I used the time alone that weekend to call Mum and Dad again and fill them in on the results of the mammogram and ultrasound. I was very much aware of how helpless they were going to feel being so far away from me, so I tried to sound as together as I could and let them know that I was coping and everything would be ok. There was still nothing definite. I explained that I now had to undergo a needle biopsy on the Monday to establish whether the lumps were benign or malignant. I told them it was probably going to be a storm in a teacup and not to worry.

I spent most of the weekend in my pyjamas and in tears, but it probably did me good to get some of it out of my system. Glenn rang as often as he could to make sure I was ok. He'd also had to explain my absence to his family, and they in turn rang with their love and support, which meant a great deal to me.

During that weekend I thought even if the worst came to the worst and I did have breast cancer, I could cope so long as I didn't have to have a mastectomy. Losing my breast was my greatest fear. It was a prospect that filled me with absolute horror. It was something I was afraid to even contemplate; if I did that, then I was accepting it might happen. It was truly my worst nightmare. I felt I could deal with anything but that. The thought of it was just too much to bear. I was reassured time and time again by the few

A FEARFUL DISCOVERY

people that knew of my situation that mastectomy was only performed in the most severe cases. It was a lifesaving measure. I might have to have a lumpectomy and some follow-up treatment, but that would probably be the extent of it.

Monday finally arrived. We had made the appointment for the needle biopsy for 2 pm which at least gave Glenn time to drive back to Cronulla on Monday morning instead of cutting his trip back home short. We drove to nearby Hurstville where I would have a blood test and the needle biopsy, which I was absolutely dreading. We were a little early for our appointment so Glenn took the opportunity to quickly pop into a shop for something he needed. I said I'd wait for him in the car and whilst I was sitting there, I decided to give Tracy a call. I'd been really careful what I'd told her until that moment as she was pregnant and I didn't want to worry or upset her. That day, I just had to call her. As soon as I heard her voice I burst into tears. I explained that I was about to have the needle biopsy and I was frightened. There were so many questions racing around my head. What if I did have cancer? What if Glenn couldn't cope and I lost him? What was I going to do? She told me not to worry, that we'd all pull together and do whatever we needed to do to beat this thing, and that she'd always be there for me, no matter what. It was exactly what I needed to hear and I was glad I'd called, though looking back now, I probably ruined her day!

By the time Glenn and I arrived at the clinic for my appointment I was extremely nervous. The doctor was very kind. Normal routine. I whipped my top off yet again and lay down on the couch whilst he administered a local anaesthetic to my left breast. Next, he inserted a fine needle into each of the lumps in my breast and withdrew a sample of cells from each. I barely felt a thing. It wasn't nearly as bad as I'd anticipated. The cells would be sent to the pathology lab for analysis and we would get the results in a day or so. All we could do now was wait.

My doctor had referred me to a surgeon, and on Wednesday, 10 September, Glenn and I had an appointment with him to discover the results of my needle biopsy.

We both sat anxiously awaiting his arrival in his rooms. The minutes ticked by. Unfortunately for us, he'd been held up in surgery that morning and was about 30 minutes late for our appointment. It felt like an eternity. He eventually arrived and beckoned us into his office. He gestured for us to take the seats opposite him and we nervously sat down. He informed us that the news was not good. The results from the needle biopsy had come back positive. I had breast cancer. I felt as if I'd been hit over the head with a sledgehammer. I thought I was going to be sick. He continued that as far as he was concerned, my only realistic course of action was to have a mastectomy. I would need chemotherapy, and that could make me infertile and even bring on early menopause. The chemotherapy would be interspersed with a five-week course of radiotherapy. I was numb. In the space of about two minutes, my whole world had come crashing down around me, my life had been turned upside down. In just one week I'd gone from not having a care in the world and being incredibly happy to being told I had cancer and could die. Glenn and I were both totally stunned. At first I could do nothing, and then the tears began rolling down my cheeks and they just wouldn't stop. I sobbed and sobbed. Glenn remained in control, although he was very shaken, and I was so glad he was there with me. There were questions that needed to be asked and I was definitely in no fit state to do that. He asked if there was any good news, any light at the end of the tunnel. All we'd been given was bad news. The surgeon said the good news was that if I had the mastectomy he could save my life.

I screamed I'd rather die than lose my breast and there was no way on earth I could agree to that operation. The thought of losing my breast was just too much for me to cope with. I'd been dreading hearing the word mastectomy. Everyone had told me I wouldn't have to have one and I'd believed them. They'd told me that women only have them now as a last resort, so was that what this was? A last resort? In a word, yes. If I didn't have the operation, then the cancer would kill me. Couldn't I have a lumpectomy instead? I could cope with that. The surgeon explained that by the time he'd performed a lumpectomy, my breast would be terribly deformed and ugly and, more importantly, there would be no guarantees that all the cancer had been removed. Sooner or later, I'd be back in to have a mastectomy anyway. I asked if I could have a reconstruction. If I could have a reconstruction, then I'd agree to the mastectomy. He said he could give me no guarantees or promises that I would be able to have a reconstruction, as it was very much dependent on the condition of my skin after radiotherapy. He didn't seem to understand why a reconstruction was so important to me. I guess it must take another woman to realise how important our breasts are to us and what an essential part of our femininity they are. There was no way I'd agree to the operation and that was that. We wanted a second opinion.

G When we took everything to the surgeon (who was 40 bloody minutes late for our appointment), he looked at the results of the biopsy and said, 'This doesn't look good' Jane was gutted. He continued: 'The test confirms you have cancer. The lumps are malignant and the only option is for you to have a mastectomy. This will be followed by radiotherapy and chemotherapy which may make you infertile. So you may not be able to have children.'

Like Jane, I just thought to myself this can't be happening. Jane, however, viewed the prognosis as a death sentence, and she lost it big time. She was scared for her life, and I was to later learn that she had good reason for feeling that way: 27 women die each day in Australia from breast cancer and one in eleven women will develop it. As for me, a bloke who has a reputation for being wild-eyed and short-tempered on the cricket field, I could do nothing but sit passively and listen to the doctor's words. He basically told Jane she had to decide whether she was prepared to lose a breast or her life. She asked if there was any chance of having a reconstruction operation; he said that would depend on the success of the operation and the way her body handled the radiotherapy and chemotherapy. Then Jane asked if she could have a lumpectomy, the process in which the tumour and surrounding breast tissue are removed and the muscle, skin and lymph nodes are left intact. However, that was not an option—it was mastectomy or death. As simple as that. To me it seemed a clear-cut choice, so I was shocked to the soles of my feet when Jane screamed that she'd rather be buried than disfigured. The doctor didn't let Jane's reaction put him off; he was relentless. I guess he had learned through his years of experience that a person sometimes has to be cruel to be kind, but watching Jane try to absorb the news was gut-wrenching stuff. Despite her howls of protest he continued; if she wanted to live, Jane would have to undergo a mastectomy followed by months of radiotherapy and chemotherapy. To get a break from the bombardment I asked whether there was any good news. The response was chilling . . . the doctor said he might be able to save her life.

What was really cruel was hearing the life-saving chemicals would pollute her bloodstream to such an extent that she could be left infertile. Jane loves kids and kids love her . . . she has a very maternal side to her and even though I had no immediate plans for a family, I could picture her with a baby in a pram and her spoiling our child rotten. It seemed the cancer was going to rob Jane of much more than her left breast.

While I tried to take in all I could, it proved a bloody hard task, because I understood very little of what the doctor said. From that experience, and from reading about the awful ritual of a doctor telling a woman of her fate, I would suggest someone accompanies a patient to the doctor's. Indeed, Lyn Swinburn, the director of National Breast Cancer Network Australia, says most women experience such a terrible shock when they're diagnosed with breast cancer that they comprehend very little of the doctor's comments so she suggests that the patient or the friend take notes to help them come to grips with the news. To be honest, I was lost when the doctor made his announcement. I didn't even know what bloody 'mastectomy' meant, but from Jane's initial reaction—absolute terror—I knew I would have to stand beside her.

In time I learnt being the partner of a woman with breast cancer is like being a corner-man for a prize fighter; no matter how badly your fighter is being mauled, you can't jump in the ring and mix it with the opponent. There were numerous times when I wished it was me suffering instead of Jane, because it would have been much easier to take. As her corner-man, all I could do was be alert and yell at my 'scrapper' to pick herself up after each body blow. It's not easy—it's a challenge which exhausts you emotionally and spiritually—but you have to 'box on'. If you don't do your job and provide support, you are taking away one of the few things the woman has to depend upon. Take my tip, helping a woman fight breast cancer is a time for selflessness and understanding.

Jane actually offered me the chance to back out of the relationship on five different occasions, saying that her health wasn't my problem. She said it was her fight and she would do it alone if need be. But I'm a firm believer that love is love. When you love someone you wear anchors, not running shoes, so there was never any chance of me deserting her. We had been together long enough for me to know Jane and I were soulmates and were meant to be together, and I had started to make serious plans for us to grow old together. I wasn't going to allow two lumps of mutant cells deny me that right, and I let her know it. I wanted to be there for Jane. I can almost understand some blokes doubting themselves and thinking perhaps they aren't up to the challenge, though. But my immediate fear was that Jane would pack her bags and return to the United Kingdom. Indeed, that thought rattled me more than the idea of tackling breast cancer head on. I couldn't imagine my life without her, and while I knew it wouldn't be a walk in the park, I was mentally prepared for anything that would be thrown my way.

While my experiences of life had lulled me into a false security about such things as cancer threats, I can honestly say that the thought of leaving didn't once cross my mind because while Jane's a striking, beautiful woman my love for her is more than skin deep. I'm head over heels in love with the whole package ... her laugh, her humour, her good cheer, her kindness, her compassion, her heart, her spirit, her love ... and that doesn't even scratch the surface. So when Jane offered me the 'escape' I told her not to be stupid; I was determined to help her every step of the way, and I'd never before been more serious

A FEARFUL DISCOVERY

about anything. There is truth in the old saying about ignorance being bliss, because while I heard the doctor talk about the risks, I didn't think for a minute that Jane could die . . . I just wouldn't believe it. While the idea of her losing a breast worried me for Jane's sake, I can say it didn't worry me as her lover. It didn't matter to me if Jane lost a breast, or even both breasts, I just wanted her to be well and here with me.

A TURNING POINT

When we arrived home after our shock diagnosis, I went into the bedroom to think about the enormity of this horrific situation. Glenn came in and sat down on the bed beside me and held me. He had been so wonderful, but I wanted to give him a way out of this nightmare. We weren't engaged or anything. He wasn't actually committed to me. This was not his problem; it was mine. I explained to him how I felt and said I would of course be flying back to England to have my treatment there. The last thing I wanted was for all of this to affect his cricket, and I definitely didn't want to be a burden to him. Most of all, I didn't want him to be with me because he felt sorry for me. If he was with me, then it had to be because he loved me, not out of pity. I said I could always return to Australia when I had completed my treatment. He wouldn't have a word of it. He told me he loved me, that we were in this together and I was going nowhere. We would beat it together. Had there been even a moment's hesitation on his part, I would have been on the next flight home.

Glenn gave Errol Alcott, the Australian team physio and a

A TURNING POINT

good friend, a call to tell him what was going on and to ask for some advice. Errol came round to the flat straight away and took a look at the mammograms for himself. Glenn mentioned to him that we wanted a second opinion and Errol telephoned his father, who is a GP. He immediately referred us to another surgeon.

The earliest appointment was for the following day, Thursday, 11 September. We drove down to the second surgeon's rooms hoping to hear some good news, that everyone had overreacted and there'd been a big mistake. Alas, it was not to be. The second opinion concurred exactly with the first—yes, I had breast cancer, yes, a mastectomy was the only option and there was even a possibility it could spread to the right breast. Just when we thought things couldn't get any worse they did with this last piece of bad news. Glenn and I were absolutely gutted. The surgeon asked if we'd like some counselling and I said yes immediately. He rang a woman who worked in this area and who could help me but she couldn't see me for a day or two—I desperately needed to see someone as soon as possible and to have to wait a day or two was too long.

I became overwhelmed by a feeling of complete helplessness, that this situation was being taken out of my hands and I was being pressured and bullied into making decisions I absolutely didn't feel ready to make. I needed to get away, quickly. Earlier in the year, Glenn had bought a property, Wancobra, 170 km northwest of Bourke, to use as a getaway, somewhere for him to have a bit of peace and quiet. It seemed like the perfect place for us to run away to, and that's exactly what I wanted to do. Glenn didn't need to be asked twice—he loves it out there. We raced back to the flat, threw some clothes into a holdall and started off on the ten-hour drive out to Wancobra. There was a wonderful feeling of relief to be leaving all of our problems behind without telling anyone where we were going. We stopped overnight at Glenn's mum's house in Dubbo (about halfway) and continued on our journey first thing the following morning. When we were about three hours away from Wancobra, we made a pit stop and popped into a small service station at a place called Byrock to buy some sweets and a couple of cool drinks. They also sold magazines, and I saw that one of them had on the front cover a story about two different women battling breast cancer. Eager for information and also inspiration, I bought it. It was a good article, but it made my predicament only too real again, and I began to wish I hadn't picked it up. I still wanted to believe there'd been a mistake and everything would be fine.

We eventually arrived at Wancobra, walked into the homestead, dumped our bags and jumped onto the motorbike for a ride around the property. It was wonderful—fresh, clean air with hundreds of emus, kangaroos and parrots all around. It was a very welcome sight after the stresses of the previous few days. Sitting on the back of the bike with my arms wrapped around Glenn's waist, I was able to forget all of my troubles and just enjoy nature's beauty around me. It was the best therapy!

G After the visit to the second specialist, it felt to Jane as if the whole world was closing in on her and she couldn't breathe. I had never witnessed a level of desperation like it before and it rocked me. Jane was searching for some light at the end of a very long tunnel and there didn't appear to be any—all she experienced in the early days of her prognosis was bad news and setbacks.

I could tell Jane needed to escape. She seemed under a tremendous amount of pressure and she needed to be detached

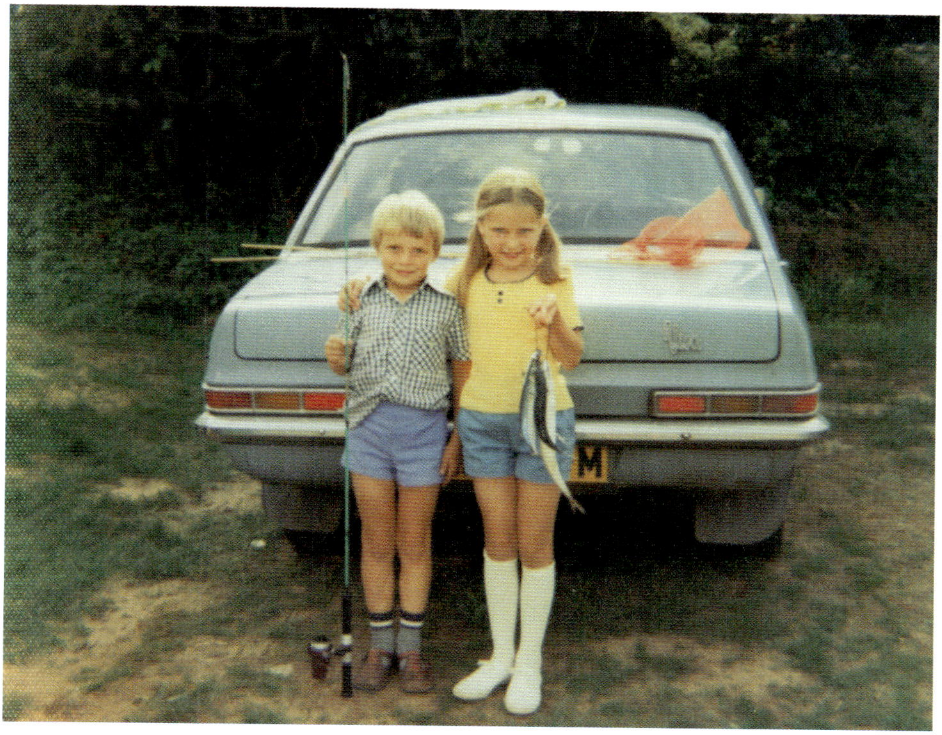

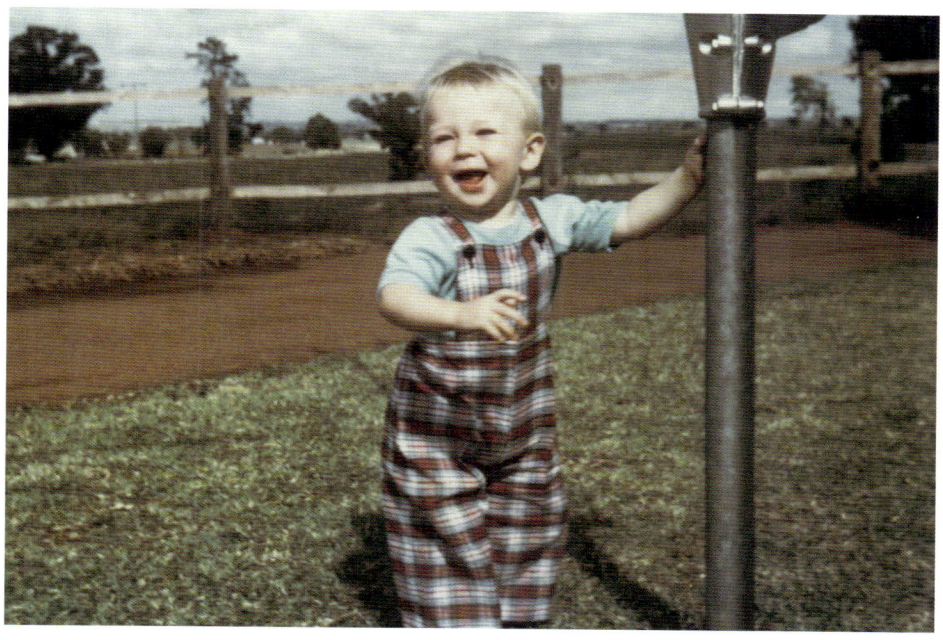

With my brother Jon in South Wales, 1974.

Glenn on the family farm, aged about two.

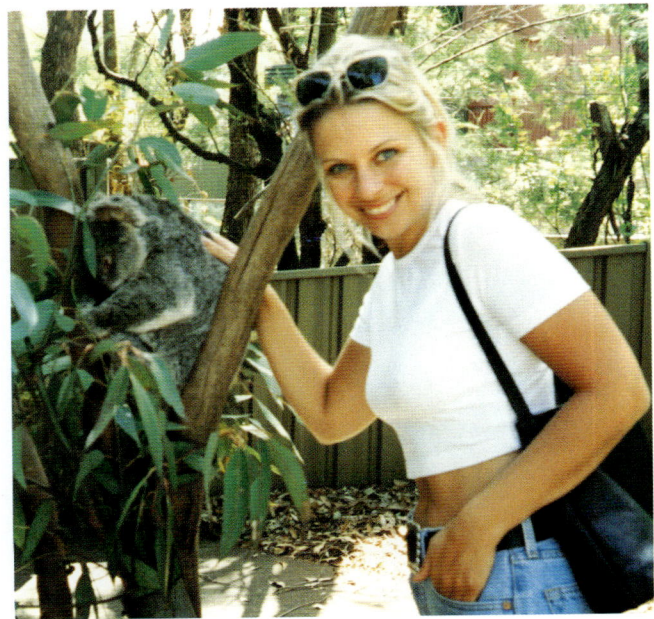

The first thing I wanted to do on my backpacking expedition Down Under was to see a koala. It doesn't look quite as thrilled as I do!

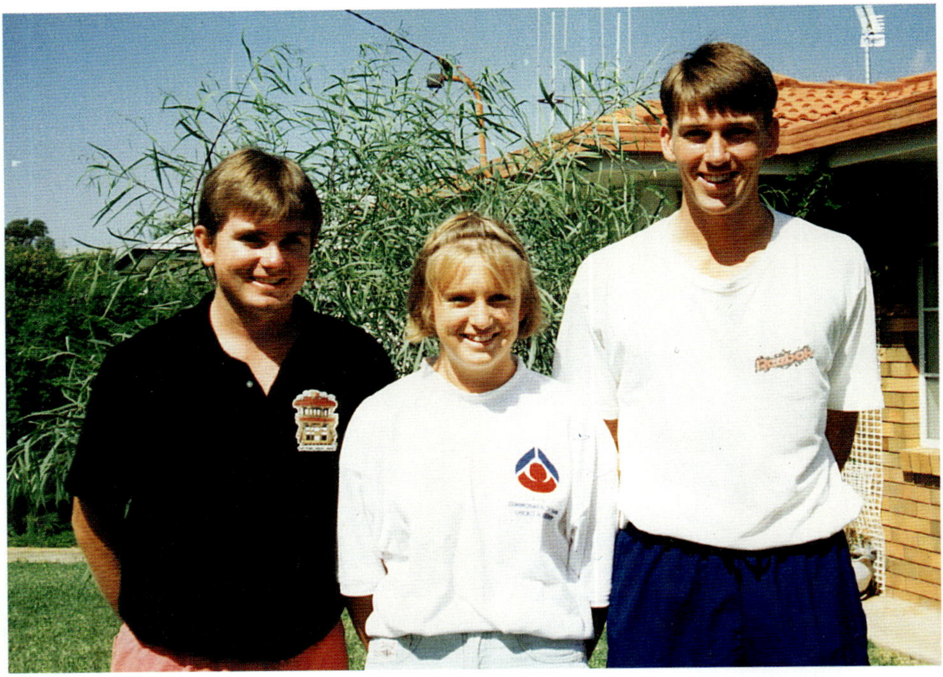

Glenn (far right) aged about twenty, with his brother Dale and sister Donna.

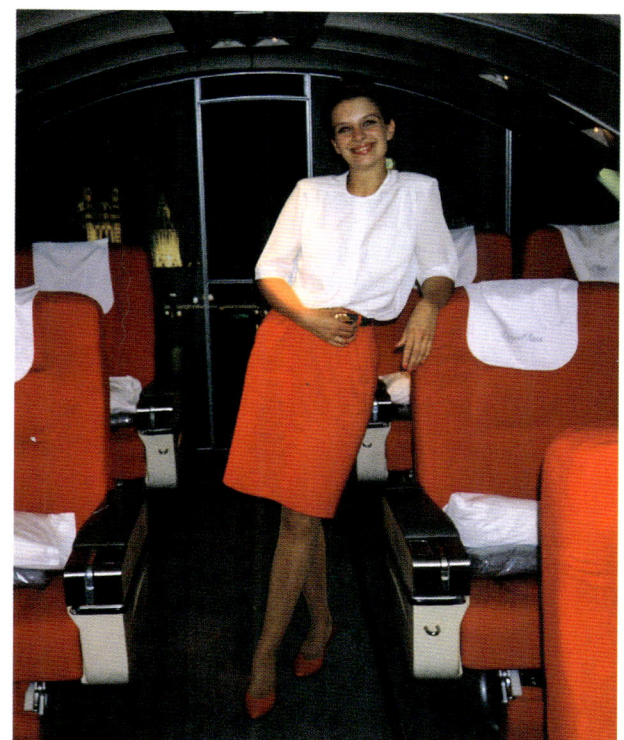

Flying high with Virgin. One of the best jobs in the world and it took me to my husband-to-be.

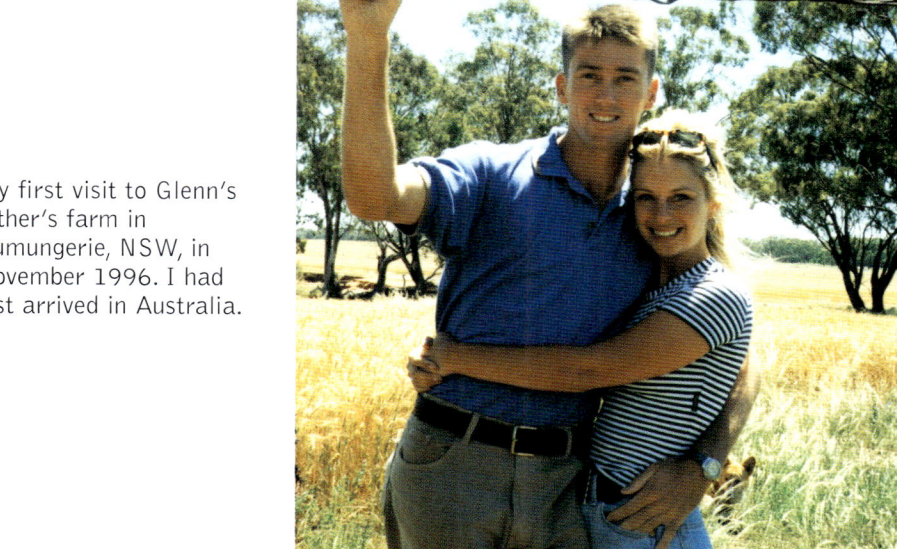

My first visit to Glenn's father's farm in Eumungerie, NSW, in November 1996. I had just arrived in Australia.

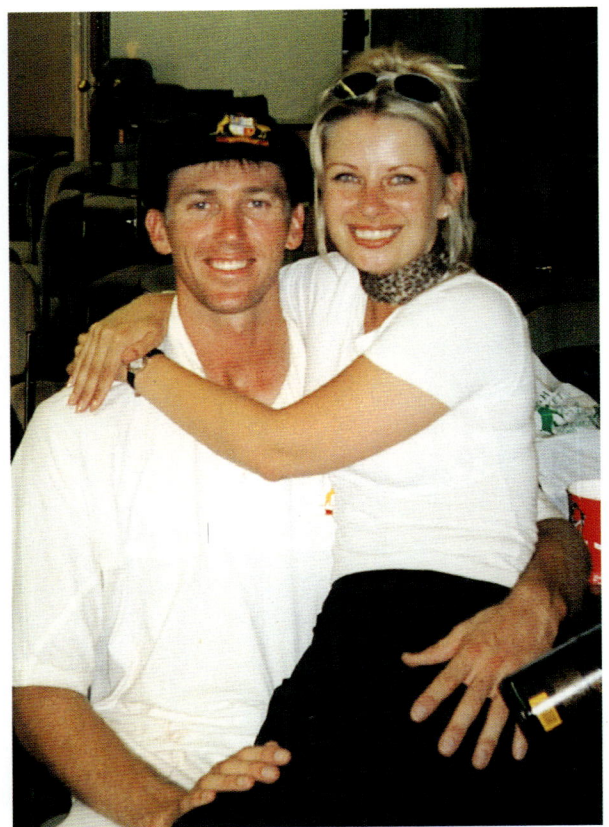

In England in 1997 celebrating after winning the Test and securing the Ashes. The lumps were there, I just hadn't discovered them.

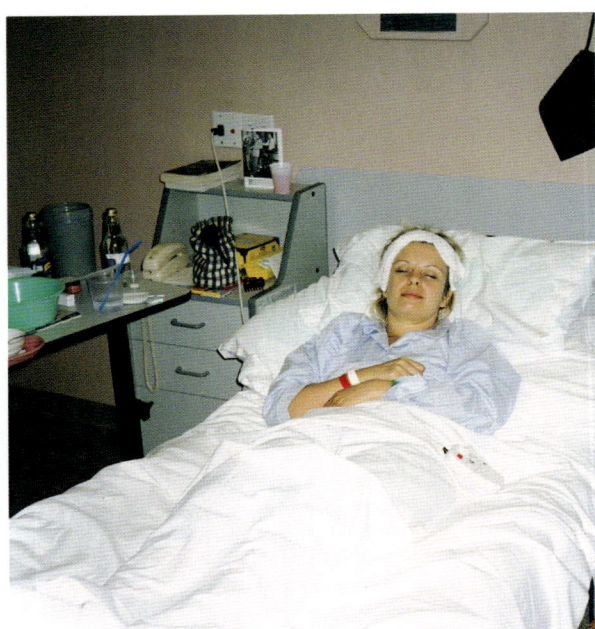

Glenn took this (unbeknown to me) shortly after my surgery, 17 September 1997.

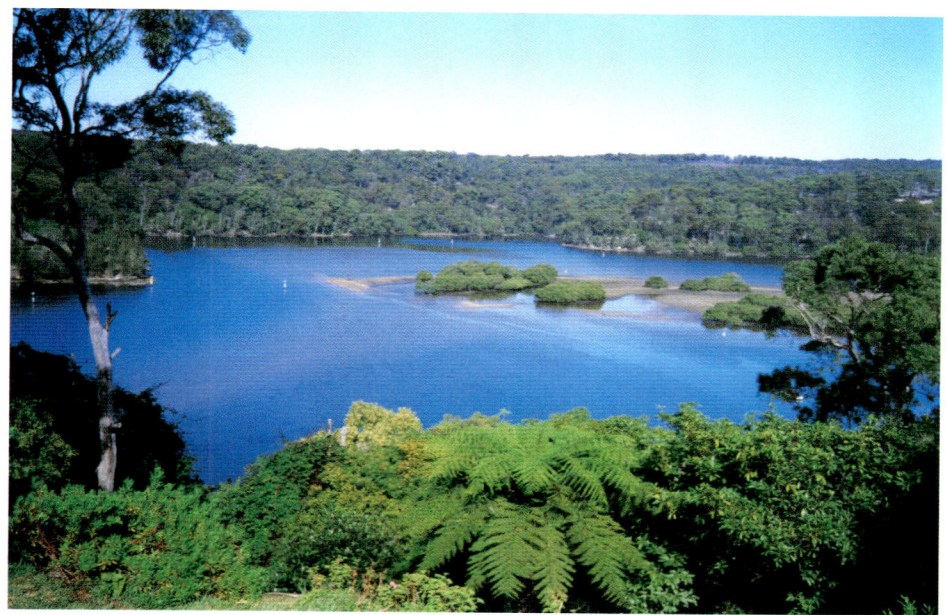

The view from our back garden in Sydney was the reason we bought the house. I gaze at this every day and thank God I'm still here to appreciate it.

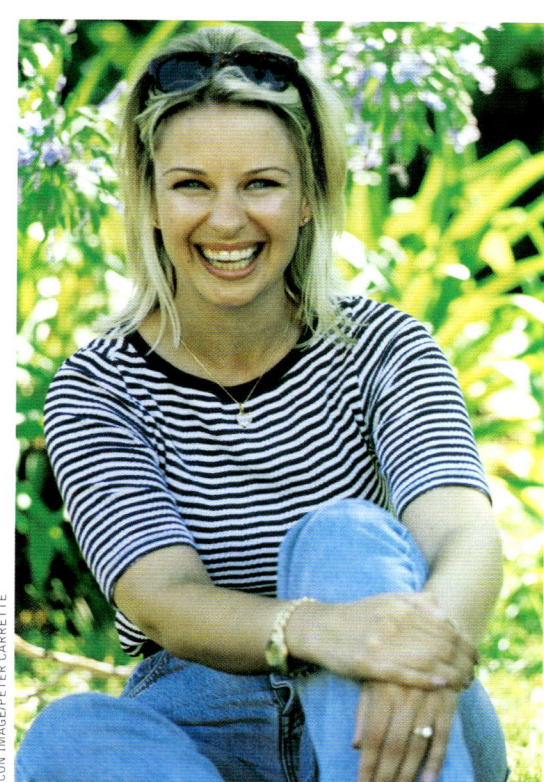

So happy! My treatment was completed and it was time for a fresh start.

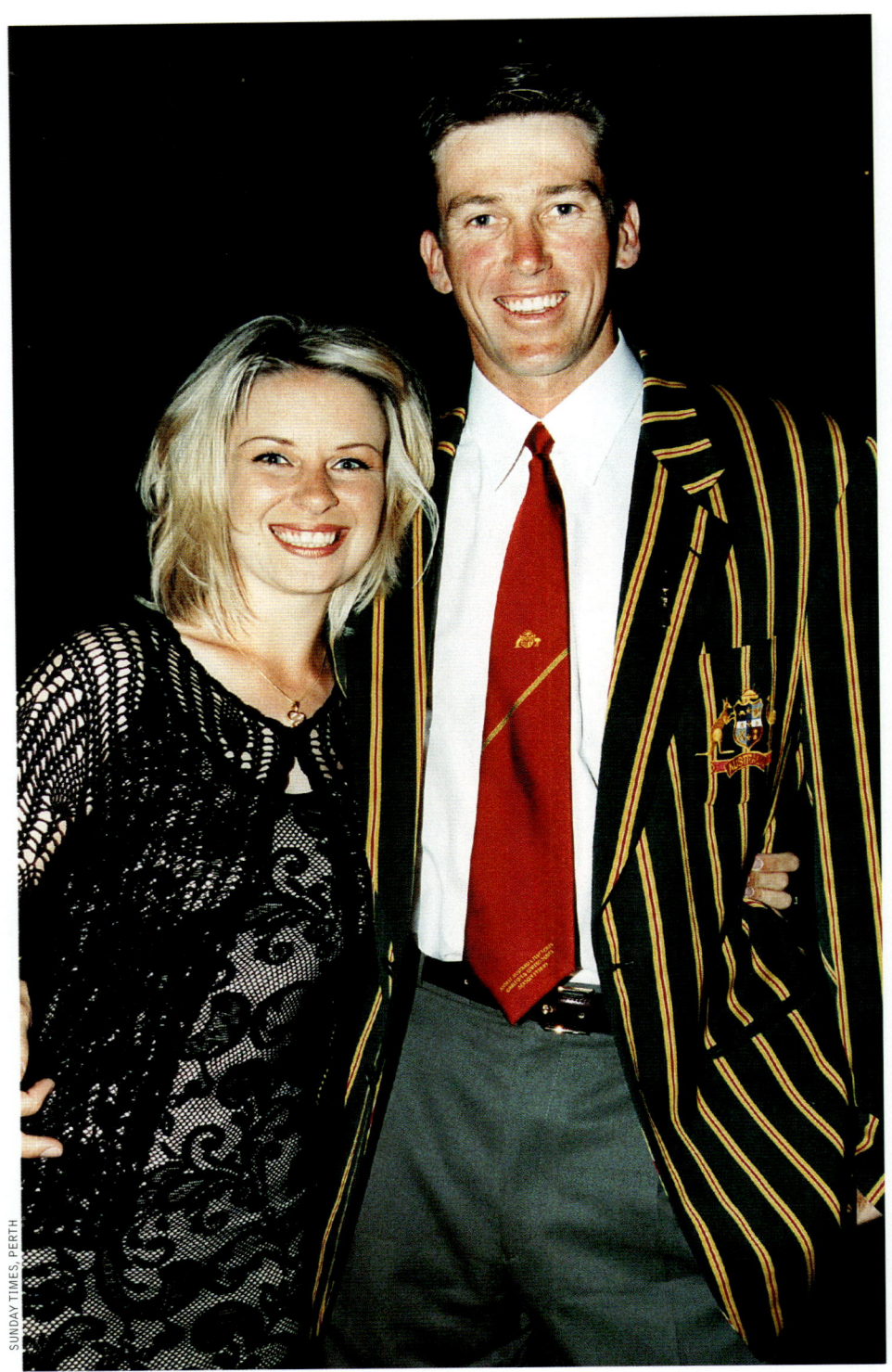

26 November 1998, Perth. Engaged!

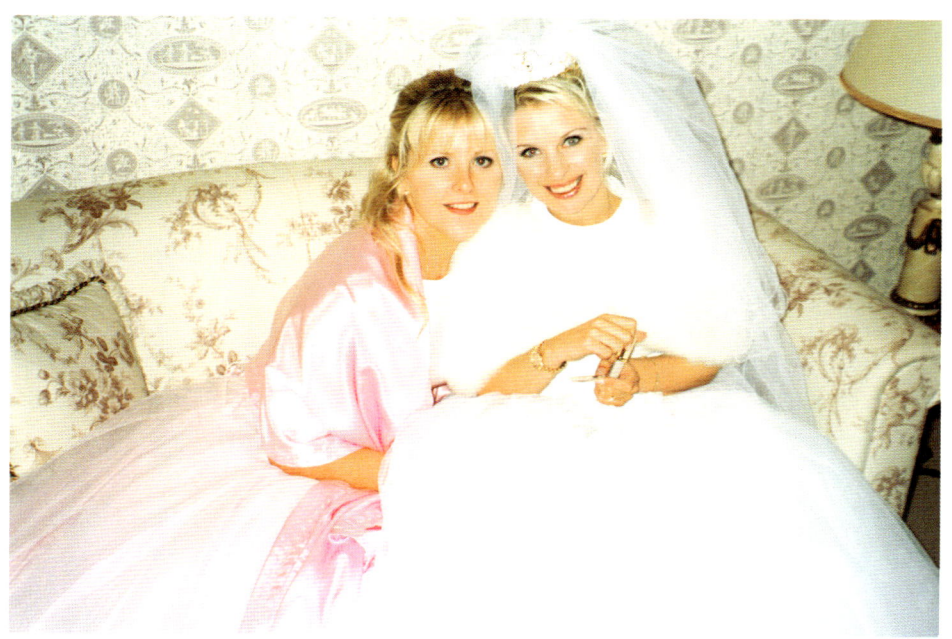

Me with Tracy Bevan. I think she was as happy as I was!

DAVID HAHN/WOMAN'S DAY

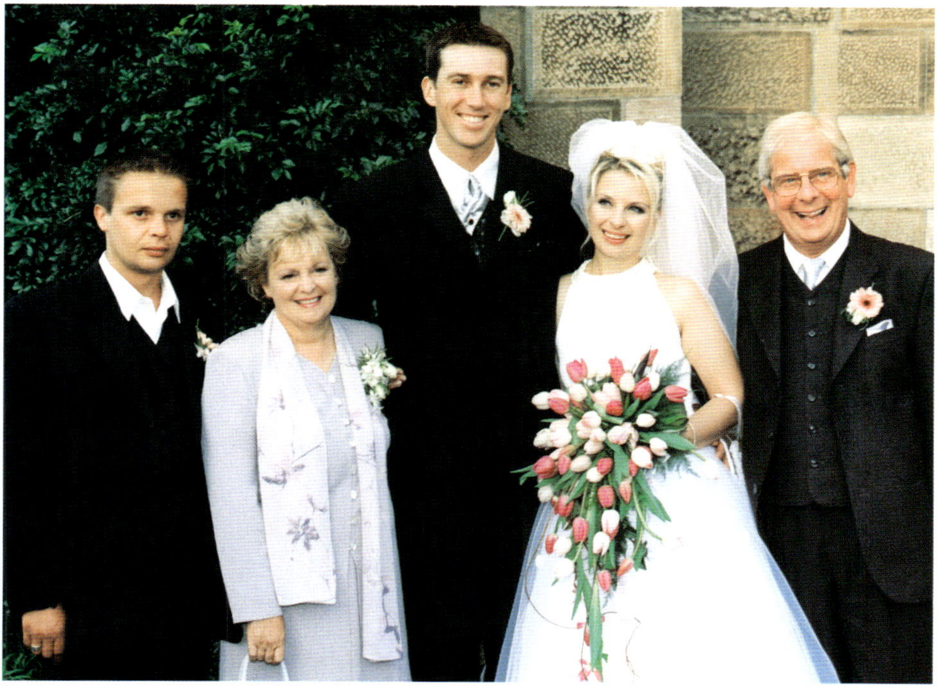

17 July 1999. The day I thought would never come. Glenn and I with my parents, Jen and Roy, and brother. Jon was feeling slightly the worse for wear from the night before but livened up in time for the reception!

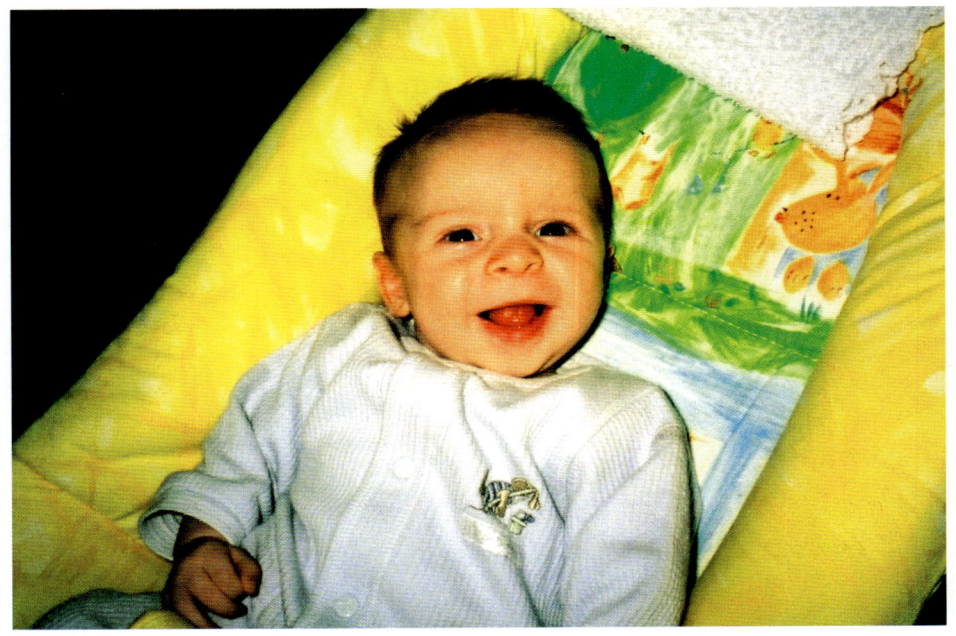

The other man in my life, our gorgeous son, James.

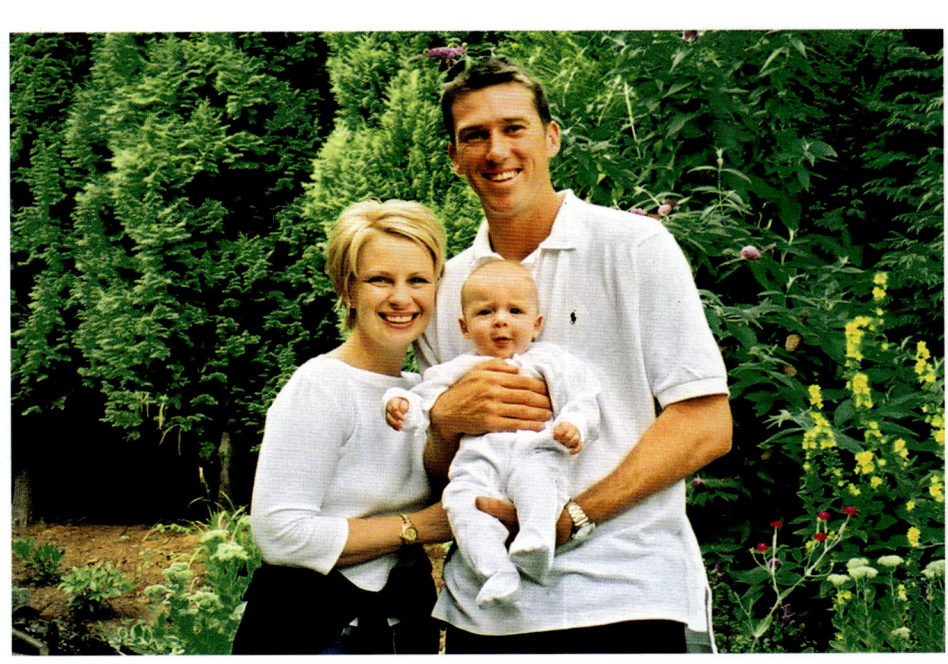

July 2000. Our family!

A TURNING POINT

from the reality of it all. My girlfriend needed a place to think more clearly and the best place I knew for that was the bush, so we loaded up the car and headed west in an attempt to find some tranquillity—and answers—on our property. While I would have given my right arm to ease Jane's pain and help her see the sense in having the operation, it turned out that she only needed to be doubled about the property on my trusty old trailbike to gain a new appreciation for life. As I have said, Jane made it painfully clear to the doctors and me that she would rather die than be disfigured, but when she saw God's grandeur—lambs, baby 'roos and emus—on two wheels and at 70 kilometres an hour, she finally realised that life is a gift to cherish, not to toss away. In the space of half a tank of petrol Jane—and I—learned to seize the day and enjoy all the magic in it. I have no doubt we're definitely better people for the lesson.

It's funny how life works, because when we returned from our trail bike ride ... our 'rebirth' ... there was a message from my skipper, Mark 'Tubby' Taylor, on the answering machine. He had heard about Jane's plight and managed to track down the number for the farm. He urged me to phone his friend Dr Chris Hughes at St Vincent's Hospital in Sydney. Tubby is one of Australia's most loved sportsmen and he uses his corporate clout for the good of a number of charities, including a group called Sporting Chance. The group raises funds for cancer research, and as a result of his involvement Mark has got to know some of the leading doctors who specialise in cancer treatment, including the amazing Dr Hughes, who was willing to talk to Jane. I phoned Chris, and his message was straight to the point. He urged Jane not to muck around with the lumps, saying it was too serious a matter. Nevertheless, he provided Jane with some much needed hope when he said if a reconstruction was all it was going to take for her to have the operation, then he would find a way to do it at a later date. He stressed that Jane's main priority was to take immediate action. His words about the reconstruction were pure gold, because when Jane had asked previously about the possibility of a reconstruction operation, the other doctors had dismissed the notion with a quick shake of the head. Dr Hughes gave her some hope, and I could see the spark flicker in her eyes when I passed on his message.

Mark will probably never know what he did for Jane and me with that one call and I'll always be indebted to my old captain for it. (Actually, one of the special things about being a member of the Australian team is the bond we members and our partners share; it is the closest thing possible to being a part of an extended family without being related by blood. The support and love we received from the likes of the Taylors, the Bevans, the Waughs and the Warnes during Jane's struggle was humbling. And it was just as moving to hear a variety of people—people we didn't even know—tell us Jane was in their prayers.)

J We'd been at Wancobra a day when Glenn received a phone call from Mark Taylor. It was Saturday, 13 September. Errol had called and told him about the breast cancer and he was ringing to offer his help and support. Mark has an involvement with the Sporting Chance Cancer Foundation, and as a result of this connection, he knows an excellent surgeon at St Vincent's Hospital. He had already called this man and informed him of our situation. The surgeon (Chris) had instructed Mark to give Glenn his number if Glenn needed anyone to talk to for help or advice. Glenn rang him straight away. I sat on the floor listening while Glenn filled Dr Chris Hughes in on all the details. He told Chris that if only I could be assured that I would be able to have a reconstruction, he was confident that I would agree to the

A TURNING POINT

mastectomy being performed. Chris replied that if that's what it would take to make me have the operation, then he would find a way for me to have it. Glenn and I were over the moon. At last, something positive, some good news—there was a glimmer of light at the end of the tunnel. I was thrilled to bits. Someone at last seemed to understand, and was on my side. I asked Glenn to call my surgeon on Monday morning and book me in for the operation. At this stage, I still couldn't even bring myself to physically say the word 'mastectomy'—it just wouldn't come out of my mouth.

Glenn went out for a bike ride, and while he was out I decided to call Mum and Dad again. They were the toughest calls I've ever had to make. Although it wasn't the news they wanted to hear, I felt that at least I had something positive to tell them. I told them that I did have breast cancer and that my surgeon had recommended that I have a mastectomy immediately. I also told them I would then have to undergo chemotherapy and radiotherapy, probably over a six-month period. I begged them not to worry, that I was going to be fine, we were lucky that we'd caught it early. I told them that I'd be able to have a reconstruction later on. Everything was going to be all right. I tried to make it sound as if I'd twisted my ankle or something. Now I'm a mother myself, I know what a completely devasting phone call it must have been for them—their only daughter was ringing them from the other side of the world to tell them she had cancer. I've discussed it with them since, and they have both told me how totally shocked they were. They just couldn't believe it could happen to me at thirty-one. I was so young. The distance made it even more difficult for them, increasing their feelings of helplessness. They were both just shattered. My brother took the news very badly. He was just stunned, and told Mum he wished it had happened to him instead. He says now that if he's ever feeling down or having a bad day, he reminds himself of what I've been through and it makes his problems pale into insignificance.

Mum consulted the support groups she already knew from her own battle with breast cancer to see what the implications were for me. She told me she had felt that something was wrong when Glenn and I were in England for the Ashes tour but didn't know what. It must have been a mother's intuition. When she found out I had detected the lump whilst in England, she was hurt that I hadn't told her about it immediately. I explained that when I first discovered the lump, it took me about two weeks to come to terms with the fact that something was very wrong. I refused to believe there might be a problem at first, and couldn't let anyone else in until I'd dealt with the prospect myself.

On Monday morning Glenn was up and out at first light, riding around the property on his motorbike again. He absolutely loves it out there. I decided to call the surgeon myself and let him know that I would have the mastectomy. They booked me in for Wednesday, 17 September. We drove back home to Cronulla that afternoon. Once I'd made the decision to go ahead and have the operation and do whatever I needed to do to stay alive, there was never any looking back. There was no feeling sorry for myself, never a 'why me?', just a strong sense of 'Right, come on let's get on with it and beat this thing'.

G When she still couldn't quite bring herself to say the word 'mastectomy', Jane viewed the tumours in her breast as a destructive force which was sucking the marrow from her life. After she came to grips with her situation Jane looked at her breast as a time bomb; she was still scared but this time it wasn't a health problem. She was fearful of losing some of her

A TURNING POINT

femininity, and, ultimately, me. She was terrified that once her operation became common knowledge there'd be women lining up to take her place alongside me. It was crazy, because they wouldn't have had a snowball's chance in hell, and I told her so constantly. We have something too special for me to just throw it away, though I know it does happen. I tried to understand where she was coming from and the best parallel I could come up with was a bloke loosing his testicles to cancer. I'm told it makes some men in this position question their manhood and fear that their partner will look elsewhere for physical fulfilment. The fear of being rejected is unfortunately one of hundreds of problems people with cancer have to address . . . but I am certain if a relationship is rock solid then it won't be a problem.

One bright light was that Jane's residency papers finally came through so she could stay in Australia. In light of the other developments, we took her residency as an omen that everything was going to be all right. Our first step to achieving that was getting Jane prepared to undergo what the doctors called a life-saving operation.

J I have always believed in fate. That everything happens for a reason, and that even though that reason may not be apparent at the time, you will come to realise why, sooner or later. Life is full of challenges, and I believe that it is the way you face up to and deal with these challenges that makes you the person you are, that makes you grow. Our lives are governed by the decisions we make for ourselves along the way. You have to take responsibility for yourself, and sometimes simply make the decision to make a decision. It's not always easy, but that's what makes life such a challenge. You can't rely on someone else to make your decisions for you and then blame them if things don't work out the way you want them to. Everyone makes mistakes along the way; as a rule, we learn from them and grow as a result. We always have the sink or swim option. It's up to us which one we choose.

I also feel that we're limited only by our own beliefs. If you think you're going to fail, chances are you will. You've thrown the towel in before you've even started. What's the point in that? Limit yourself and you will be limited. If you don't believe in yourself, why should anyone else? The mind is an extremely powerful tool and we should use it to our advantage, not let it hinder or restrict us. I believe that positive thinking is a tremendous weapon in conquering the battle against illness and disease. When you're feeling at your lowest ebb, never lose sight of your goals and never underestimate your inner strength. Believe in yourself. It's amazing what you can achieve when you put your mind to it.

When you're diagnosed with breast cancer, or any life-threatening illness, it doesn't affect just you—it affects everyone around you as well. It really helped me knowing that my family and friends were there fighting with me every step of the way. Their support was absolutely invaluable. The cards, letters, flowers and phone calls meant so much to me. They brightened my days and lifted my spirit. I always felt it must be harder for them sitting on the sidelines, having to stand by and watch me do the hard yards; I was just getting on with it and doing what I had to the best way I knew how. I actually liken it to watching Glenn playing cricket. I bowl every ball and face every batsman with him but have no control over the outcome, and I think this is probably more stressful than actually being him and just getting on with the job at hand!

During this time Glenn's family would ring from the country to see how I was and to tell me that people I'd never even met who knew of my plight were sending their love and saying prayers for me. I found all this extremely comforting, even though I'm not especially religious. It helped immensely knowing I was surrounded by so much love and support.

Another important factor for me was that I also wanted Glenn to be proud of me. He had shown me his love was unconditional and I was determined not to let him down.

I sometimes felt that maybe I had been chosen to get breast cancer because I was strong enough to fight it, to take it on and beat it. That maybe other women in a similar position would then see that having breast cancer isn't necessarily a death sentence—that they could win their battle too. If I'd done it, so could they. That might sound a bit bizarre, but it gave me another reason to get through it all. As I said earlier, the mind is a very powerful thing.

BLACKEST DAYS

J Looking back, I think that my blackest days fell between being diagnosed with breast cancer on Wednesday, 10 September and actually going into hospital for the mastectomy on Wednesday, 17 September. I remember being in an absolute state of shock at how quickly your perfect little world can come tumbling down around you. One day you are the happiest girl on earth, without a care in the world. The next you hear your name followed by the word cancer and suddenly there's a chance that it could all be over, just like that. No warning. It came as such a shock. I'd never been happier and I felt great, as fit as a fiddle, and then I'm told, completely out of the blue, that I'm dying on the inside. It must be the most incredible drop from high to low ever. I thought about some of the things I'd worried about and agonised over pre-diagnosis. Now those same problems were of no consequence whatsoever, they meant absolutely nothing. Having breast cancer instantly put my whole life into perspective. Every morning I'd wake, get up and walk into the bathroom to take a shower. I'd undress down to my waist and stand in front of the bathroom mirror just gazing at my left breast. Instead of seeing my own reflection, all I could see was the ugliness of the cancer inside, eating me away. I knew it would kill me if I didn't do something quickly to stop it, and I hated it. Once I had made the decision to go ahead with the mastectomy, these feelings of hate only intensified, and from that moment on, I *never* looked back.

After driving home from Wancobra, Glenn and I went to the hospital on the afternoon of 16 September to complete the necessary pre-admission forms. After completing the relevant paperwork, the receptionist offered to show me to my room. She had assumed I was there to 'check in' for my surgery the following day. I was overwhelmed by a feeling of panic. I wasn't ready yet, and hadn't been expecting to have to stay that night in hospital. I needed to have that last night at home with Glenn. We'd planned to go out for dinner at one of our favourite restaurants and I was so looking forward to it. I asked if there was any way I could be admitted the next morning instead. She told us we'd have to be at the hospital really early and not to have anything to eat for breakfast. I didn't need telling twice. We were out of there, quick as a flash.

We returned to the hospital early the next morning and were shown to the room where I'd be staying. I was one of the first patients on my surgeon's list that morning, which meant that I didn't have a long wait. I was grateful for that. Glenn and I just sat on the bed watching some television—I think Bert Newton might have been on but it's all a bit of a blur. I was extremely apprehensive. I knew that this operation was going to change my life forever and that some of those changes would take quite a bit of getting used to. I was also trying to put myself in Glenn's shoes, wondering how he was feeling. If he was worried or concerned about my wellbeing or our future, he didn't show it once, not once. All I felt was the warmth of his love and his unwavering support.

The nurse came in and gave me a gown to wear and a pair of those super paper pants. I always remember a girlfriend telling me about the time she had to go into hospital and was told to strip down to her knickers and put a gown on. It was a gown that fastened at the back with a tie at the top—there were no other fasteners. Unfortunately for her, she had worn a g-string that day, not giving her hospital appointment a second thought. Mortified at the thought of her bottom being exposed to all and sundry, she asked the nurse for a pair of paper pants and was told that they'd run out. In a panic, she sent her husband dashing off to a nearby Marks & Spencers to buy her a pair of 'big' pants. By the time he returned it was too late and she'd already had to leave for her operation, desperately trying to hold the back of her gown together. I'd remembered her telling me that story and had worn 'big' knickers that day, just in case my hospital had a shortage of paper pants!

It seemed like no time before they came to wheel me down for surgery. All of a sudden I felt incredibly frightened. Glenn walked with me for as far as he was allowed, and held my hand the whole way. I didn't want to let him go. It must have been so hard for him, seeing me lying there sobbing and knowing there was nothing more that he could do. We both knew I had to have the operation, but even with the reality of it staring us in the face, I don't think either of us could quite believe it. When he had to leave me, I became extremely upset, and succeeded in working myself up into a real state. My friend Bev was working at the hospital that day and she was called to come and attempt to calm me down. The anaesthetist was angry with the nurses taking care of me for somehow overlooking my pre-med. As a result, I was extremely upset and very agitated—not an ideal state for pre surgery.

I have an allergic reaction to Amoxil and so for my operation, instead of wearing a normal white hat to cover my hair, I had to wear a red one to indicate the allergy. My final humiliation came as I lay there waiting to go in for surgery, with Bev trying to calm me down. There were two male patients, who I think must have been waiting in recovery. I remember them seeing me lying there with my red hat on and tears rolling down my cheeks. I heard them make a joke about the red hat and start laughing. Looking back now, I can't believe they could have been so insensitive. My tears just wouldn't stop.

G When Jane had finally consented to the operation the surgeons had made immediate arrangements for her to be admitted to the Kareena Private Hospital. It's only in hindsight that I truly appreciate that their haste was because we were dicing with a lot more than mere cosmetic surgery. It was life and death.

The private hospital arrangement meant that it did cost quite a lot in the end, more than $4000, and one worry which haunted Jane from the earliest days of her battle was not having any private health insurance in Australia. She was terrified by the amount the procedures would cost. Unfortunately, that is a very real fear for thousands of the people who are faced with long-term medical treatment. From my end, at least, I can say the money involved in helping Jane was never going to be an issue. I'm the first to admit that as a professional sportsman I am better off than the average, but I can assure you, had I needed to dig ditches or work as a brickies' labourer in my spare time to ensure that the operation and other treatments were paid for, I would have done so—and gladly.

On her arrival at the hospital Jane was tense and nervous, and it was one of the rare times where it was impossible for me to dismiss the gravity of the situation with a trademark 'no worries' wave of my bowling hand. The best I could do to try to help ease Jane's fear was to tell her I understood, that I loved her, and that I'd be with her every step of the way. Apart from that there were few other words that could help, because in just a matter of hours we both knew Jane was going to lose her breast—and unlike the movies, where a miracle cure is found at the last minute, we knew nothing could change her immediate fate. But our acceptance of the necessity of the operation meant we had some control over what seemed at times to be an uncontrollable situation. That acceptance helped us to learn how her cancer affected us. While we were dealing with a very serious matter Jane's more positive frame of mind allowed us to 'breathe'. In the early days of Jane's prognosis I read all I could on the illness in the belief that to be forewarned is to be forearmed. The material I read was anything but light . . . it was pitch black, with statistics and personal accounts painting a terrifying portrait: In 1997 in Australia 10,000 women were diagnosed with breast cancer—that works out to be 27 each day, and in the same year 2500 died as a result of the disease— that's an average of one woman every four hours. Also: one in eleven women will develop breast cancer; the risk of dying is seventeen times greater if it isn't detected early, while it is still in only the breast; women aged over 40 should have a regular mammogram—every two years; and women of all ages should self-examine each month and have an annual GP check-up.

While Jane's anguish before the operation distressed me deeply, I knew that no matter what her breast looked like after the doctors finished their work it would not affect my feelings towards her. Nothing could. She would still walk the same, smell the same, laugh the same, cry the same and rather than mourn her impending change of figure I actually rejoiced within. That might sound strange to some people, but I rejoiced because I dared to believe that the operation was going to allow us a bloody good chance to ring in our old age together. Our future was all that mattered to me. I tried not to allow any negative thoughts to settle in my mind in the lead-up to the operation. Instead I steeled my nerves by telling myself that if Jane could deal with the situation, then I could too. I took a leaf out of Jane's book—I expelled any negative thoughts and embraced the positive ones. Courage, and not tears, were needed from my end. While I never thought I would collapse, I sensed that if I did cave in it would have had a devastating affect on her.

I've heard people say from time to time that what I do on the cricket field is brave, but believe me, it's not. Playing professional cricket is a job (and a great one at that) and I choose to do it. However, in the reality stakes, if I make a mistake, it isn't then the end of the world. If a batsman whacks a six off my bowling—even in a one-day match—I get a shot at redemption with the next ball; if a fieldsman drops a catch off my bowling, I return to my mark and try all over again; if Australia loses a match, well, the sun still rises the next day and we get on with life despite the headlines. Jane's illness showed me another side of life, and led me to believe that the word 'courageous' is bandied about far too easily. When it's all said and done, the real heroes are those people who try to ignore their pain and crack a joke long after they've forgotten what feeling 'normal' is like; they're the parents and partners of ill people—mental or physical—who fight on against devastating odds; they're the doctors and the scientists working around the clock trying to find a cure to the diseases which cause heartache on a daily basis. My main hero in life is Jane and the way in which she survived her ordeal through her strength; her attitude and character means she'll always be my idol.

I walked with Jane for as long as I could until they wheeled her into surgery and I recall a bright red cap being placed on her head. Unfortunately, she thought two blokes in the hallway were laughing at the sight of her. Naturally enough Jane was already in a fragile state, and the sound of their guffaws sent her into hysterics. Her outburst was so bad the orderlies were asked to track down our friend Bev Mitchell from another part of the hospital to try and help calm her down.

It was awful sitting alone with my thoughts while Jane was being operated on a few rooms away. While we were separated by solid walls, I was with her in spirit and I felt her pain . . . every last ounce of it. Her room was crammed with bunches of flowers sent by a number of well-wishers, and I took comfort in seeing their colours because I knew Jane would be happy to see them once she woke. As I watched Jane in her post-operative sleep I felt as if I was looking at the face of one of life's real scrappers. I couldn't help but feel sad, though, because I knew that while she'd fought—and fought hard—for her life, she had an even rougher battle ahead with chemotherapy and radiotherapy. Jane had her gown on but I could tell her chest was swathed in bandages and dressings.

J The next thing I recall is waking up back in my room with Glenn sitting by my bedside. He was a wonderful sight. I was in a real daze and still can't remember too much about this period. I wasn't in any pain and there was no soreness, probably because I was pumped full of pethidine. Bev was still on shift, and she stopped by to see how I was. She explained that I had a button by my bed which would administer more pethidine if I needed it when I pressed it. I remember pressing it, without actually being aware of what

I was doing. I definitely couldn't feel any pain! By the end of the day, my room was filled with so many beautiful flowers they had to be taken out of my room so that I could sleep—their perfume was too strong. I was overwhelmed by the kindness and support of family and friends once again.

The next morning, I woke up and felt good. The nurse came and helped me to shower. I was a bit stiff and the two drains in the left-hand side of my chest made movement a bit awkward but I managed. After freshening up, I sat up in bed and put all my make-up on. I wanted to look good for when Glenn arrived. I wanted him to see I was coping. The surgeon came in to see how I was. I think he was somewhat surprised to see me sitting up in bed, full make-up on looking more like a visitor than a patient. Obviously, the painkillers were doing a great job. In fact my only discomfort was from the drains. The drains were there to empty the fluid from my wound. I could see that there was a yellow liquid filling the tubes—the sight of it made me feel physically ill. I hated having the drains in. If I moved in a certain way, they felt like needles sticking into me. I also hated the thought of having a foreign plastic tube inside my body; together with the sight of them, this also made me feel extremely sick. By the time I could have one of them removed, about four days after the surgery, I had worked myself up into quite a state about them, and was absolutely dreading having them taken out. In the end, the nurse offered me a couple of valium, which I gratefully accepted . . . the whole thing became a blur.

During my stay in hospital following the mastectomy, I was very heavily bandaged. When I found myself alone (which wasn't very often, as Glenn was there every day and night), I would run my fingers over the dressings on the area where the breast had been, to see what it felt like. I knew that the whole breast had been removed, but the more I felt, the more I was sure that where the breast had been was actually now concave. My imagination began to run riot. I was terrified that there would be a gaping hollow on the left-hand side of my chest. I didn't tell Glenn—I thought he might run a mile if I did. During the mastectomy, the surgeon had also taken a sample of lymph nodes from under my left arm. They do this in order to tell whether and how far the cancer has spread, as the lymph nodes in the axilla (armpit) are usually the first place that breast cancer spreads to. Lymph nodes are tiny kidney-shaped sacs that get rid of bacteria and other waste products. The main ones are found in the neck, axilla and groin. The number of lymph nodes removed depends on how many are in the tissue that is removed from the armpit. In my case, there were twenty lymph nodes taken and two of these were found to be cancerous. Fortunately for me, they were the two closest to my left breast, which meant that the cancer had probably been caught in the nick of time. But this also meant that the mastectomy scar extended across the left-hand side of my chest and up into my left armpit, which resulted in the movement in my left arm being extremely limited following the operation. I would need to do a lot of physio to get full movement and use back into my arm.

I hated being in hospital and was desperate to go home. My surgeon told me that when I could put my hands on my head, he would allow me to go home. Every day I did the exercises I'd been shown, but moving my arm was very painful. It felt like a lead weight. I wondered if I would ever have full, normal use of it again. I am left-handed, so I was probably using it more than I would have had it been my right arm that had been affected.

On day five of my stay in hospital, it was time to take off the bandages. I asked Glenn to leave the room while the surgeon examined the scar and surrounding area. He was pleased with the way it was all healing and asked if I was ready to look at the scar. Before the operation I had declared that I would only ever look at my scar when I had to, and vowed that Glenn would never see it. But my surgeon felt it was very important that I see the scar before I went home. He felt that it was important for Glenn to see it as well. I was absolutely horrified. I'd already told Glenn he would never see it. We'd agreed. What if he took one look and passed out? What if he thought it was so ugly he couldn't bear to be near me any more? The surgeon felt that Glenn should decide for himself, and called him back into the room. Never mind Glenn being ready to see the scar—I didn't even know if I was ready! Finally I reluctantly agreed. After all, if it meant I could go home, it would all be worth it. I had already been able to put my hands on my head for the surgeon. I was having a good day. Glenn admitted that yes, he would like to see the scar. I thought of the gaping hollow I'd envisaged and my heart sank. The moment of truth had arrived. I resigned myself to getting it over and done with. If he can't cope with it, then it's better I find out now rather than later, I thought.

My heart was pounding so hard as the dressings were slowly removed. Glenn was standing in front of me as I sat perched on the edge of the hospital bed. I don't know which one of us was the more nervous. Finally, all the bandages were off and the surgeon told me to look down. Glenn had looked and he was still standing, so I thought it couldn't be that bad. I took a deep breath and gingerly looked down. It wasn't concave at all, thank goodness. In fact, I have to say that given the dramatics of my imagination, I was pleasantly surprised. The area where the breast had been was just flat, with a line of staples across the scar, which was about fifteen centimetres long. I could cope with that. One of the most amazing things I noticed was that I could see the skin rising and falling where my heart was beating beneath it. I'd felt my heart beat, of course, but never actually seen it. It was a great sight! Glenn did not appear to be fazed one bit. I've asked him since whether he was, but he still maintains that it didn't bother him. The even better news was that I could now go home.

G Jane's first look at the scar was always going to be tough. She had made it clear before the operation that she didn't intend for me to see it—ever. The doctor told Jane he thought it would be best for me to take a look before she was discharged from hospital. I'm being sincere when I say the result was nowhere near as bad as Jane had feared. There was no hollow dent; it was a clean, neat scar. It didn't repulse me as Jane had thought it would . . . I didn't feel queasy, and I didn't feel the need to run for the hills. Instead, all I could do was marvel at how good a job the doctor had done. Even now, a few years down the track, when I look at that scar I think of it as Jane's badge of courage. Actually, like other women who lose a breast to cancer, Jane is now an Amazon, just like the tribe of women from Greek mythology. According to the ancient Greeks, the women warriors would cut a breast off so that they could fire their arrows without any hindrance. As I say, Jane is courageous, and that scar also represents a time when she realised life was worth living no matter what. I honestly can't see how any man would find such a thing ugly. It's not only a constant reminder of my love for her but it also prompts me to take nothing in life for granted.

J As I said, once I'd made my decision to proceed with the mastectomy, I never looked back. Although it was an extremely difficult decision for me to make at that time, I knew deep down in my heart that it was the only one. I would rather be living a full life with one breast than be six foot under with two—there's no contest there! It's hard to believe now that I ever said I would rather be dead than lose my breast, but I guess saying it was a true indication of just how devastated and shocked I was at the time. I could not believe it was all happening. It's also funny looking back and remembering how I said adamantly that I would never look at my scar and that Glenn would most definitely never ever see it. Now, it doesn't bother me in the slightest. In fact, I look at my scar every morning and evening and I thank God it's there, because if it wasn't, then I wouldn't be either. Don't get me wrong, of course I'd prefer to look in the mirror and see a pair of beautiful healthy breasts (who wouldn't!), which is why I'm planning a reconstruction in the not too distant future. I'm hoping they'll give the right breast a little nip and tuck as well, and I'll end up looking better than ever. I guess what I'm trying to say is that when I look at my scar, it's not something that ever makes me depressed, or makes me think 'Why me?' Not once have I asked 'Why me?' It's not a question that ever entered my head. Feeling negative like that is going to get you nowhere fast. I believe you should take the time to grieve for your breast if you feel the need to, but then you simply have to get on with your life. Life is too short to be bitter and full of resentment. You'll only succeed in bringing yourself down and stretching out your recovery. I have *never* viewed my mastectomy as a mutilation of my body; quite the opposite, actually. I see my scar as a celebration of my winning my battle against breast cancer, and I thank my lucky stars for it. It's now as much a part of me as everything else I was fortunate enough to be born with.

G While I think she looks great as she is, Jane is still keen to have her breast reconstruction. However, I have told her to do that for herself and not me. It won't bother me in the slightest if she decides not to go ahead with the procedure—like everything else involved with breast cancer, the plastic surgery required for a reconstruction is laced with pain and some (slight) risks. Surgeons have to cut a patient open again, remove muscles and use them to build up the breast before performing skin grafts. The reconstruction is something I would like for Jane to go into more thoroughly because from trawling the internet my understanding of the procedure is while there's a healthy success rate there is also some risk of complications including bleeding, infection, bad scars, loss of feeling in the arm or hand, drug and anaesthetic reactions up to and including death (though I must stress that's rare). Nevertheless, those facts mean any operation is something we must talk about at much greater length because I really want Jane to understand that she doesn't have to endure the procedure in the mistaken belief she needs to do it in order for me to be happy. Believe me, I couldn't be happier with her.

J The day I was allowed to go home, Glenn had a meeting with a sponsor up in Brisbane. He offered to cancel it, but I insisted he go. I was determined that our lives would not change, and that we should try to lead as normal a life as possible. He was able to take me home from hospital, but then he had to leave for the airport straight away. Our friend Bev came round to the flat to make sure I was alright and to see if I needed anything. She and Darren stayed the night with me so that I wouldn't be alone on my first night at home.

The next day I realised that no one would have been to collect our mail from our post office box down in Cronulla and I asked Bev if she'd mind running me down there quickly before she went off for her round of golf. She tried to talk me out of it but I insisted. I checked my reflection in the mirror before leaving, and realised, to my horror, that my chest was lopsided. I hadn't even thought of this. What was I going to do? No one had given me any advice on what happens post-mastectomy, or on prostheses. I knew absolutely nothing. I decided to put a pair of socks there instead, but as I was unable to wear a bra because of the bandages, there was nowhere to put them. I began to get very angry, and wondered what was I going to do, not just about going down to collect the post but for the rest of my life. I just wanted to look normal. In the end, I threw on my leather jacket and hid myself away underneath it and off we went. By the time we drove into Cronulla, which was only about five minutes from our home, I was feeling very weak, but I was still determined to get the mail. I don't know why. It was just important to me to go and get it. I guess it was just part of my desire that my life shouldn't be any different because of my operation. As Bev parked the car and we walked to the post office, I felt as though I had the word 'mastectomy' tattooed across my forehead. I was sure the whole world knew that I only had one breast now. We grabbed the mail and Bev drove me back home. I was exhausted. It was my first taste of real life after the operation, and I knew it was going to be a tough ride.

Glenn rang from Brisbane later that day to see how I was going. I told him I was fine and asked how he was. He told me he'd had quite a big night and was still feeling slightly the worse for wear. He'd gone out with Craig McDermott and a couple of his sponsors and got through what sounded like a whole bottle of Jack Daniels. He'd had a speaking engagement that morning and had to keep excusing himself to go and be sick! This was not like Glenn. The Glenn I knew didn't get drunk. A few beers with the boys and a night out after a win, of course, but that was about it. I panicked. I took it as a sign that he had been putting on a brave face with me all along, when the reality was that he couldn't cope with the situation we'd suddenly found ourselves in at all. The first time he's away from me, he goes out and gets absolutely smashed. This was not good. I didn't say anything to him on the phone, but Bev was with me when I'd taken the call and I told her about what had happened. She said I was over-reacting, which I probably was, but it was just so out of character for Glenn. Whenever he has to go to Brisbane now, there's a standing joke between us about him painting the town red while he's up there!

Due to the limitation of movement with my left arm, I was unable to bathe myself or wash my hair for a day or so, and once again, with Glenn up in Brisbane, Bev came to the rescue. I felt like a child. I was so helpless and reliant on Bev and Glenn, and I hated it. I'd been out of hospital for three days before I could shower and wash my hair by myself—it felt great, if a little awkward! Although I am a very independent person, I'm not too proud to ask for help when I need it, and I was—and still am—very grateful that I had friends nearby who cared. I was still unable to drive or do much physically. As Glenn was going to be away on and off for a few weeks, we decided to ask my mum to fly out and stay with us for a little while. Why is it that you always seem to want your mum when you're not feeling well? She came out for a couple of weeks, which was great. As my recovery was going so well, she ended up flying back to England a week earlier than expected! One evening we were sitting on the settee watching television and I turned to her and asked if life would ever feel normal again. All I could think about was the course of treatment that lay ahead of me and the possibility that the cancer could come back. I suppose it's quite natural to think about those things when you've so recently had surgery for breast cancer. All your thoughts are consumed with it and you think of little else. Mum smiled and said that yes, all those thoughts and feelings do pass, but it takes time. And she was right, they did pass and yes, life does go back to normal, but it's never quite the same as it was before—it's even better. For me, the sky is always a little bit bluer and the birds sing just that little bit more sweetly. I appreciate the little things in life, the simple things, so much more—they're the things that are important to me now. I feel I've had an insight into just how precious they are. I think it's quite sad that most people go through their lives not even noticing them. I feel I'm lucky to see things this way and my life is much richer because of it.

I had left hospital with no information on my life, indeed my body, post-mastectomy. No phone numbers of organisations that could help me or offer me support, nothing. Once again, it was my friend Bev who rang the Cancer Council on my behalf and explained my situation to them. They were wonderful, and immediately sent me out a 'softie', together with a breast cancer information pack. The 'softie' was made of a filling similar to cushion stuffing and packed into a silky pouch which just slips into your bra. It was wonderful to have a 'breast' again—at least to the outside world, I would look normal. I was thrilled with this development and thought I handled my softie pretty well, still wearing the tight lycra tops I used to wear before the operation. One evening a couple of weeks after my operation, Glenn had been invited as a guest on the Roy & HG show *Club Buggery*, and I went along with Glenn and his manager, Warren Craig, to watch. It was my first night out with my softie. I wore tight black trousers and a thigh-length black jacket with a crimson shirt underneath. Warren and I were in the front row of the studio audience, so we had a great view of proceedings. Glenn came out and the interview began. It was going really well. I suddenly felt a little uneasy, and a small flash of cream silk just below my line of vision caught my eye. I glanced down only to see my softie poking out of the top of my jacket—I nearly died! Fortunately for me, no one else had noticed—they'd probably have thought it was a hanky or something if they had spotted it. Anyway, I tried to nonchalantly shove it back down into my bra before anyone saw. After that experience, I always used safety pins to secure it in place before venturing out in public.

It was clearly time for me to get a prosthesis. I was pleasantly surprised to learn that I could be fitted for one at a nearby Grace Bros store in the lingerie department. They had a private changing room dedicated to fitting prostheses and trained staff available to fit them. (Not every store has this facility so it's best to ring to find the one closest to you.)

There is a wide variety of breast forms to choose from, in many shapes and sizes depending on the type of surgery you've had. There is something to suit everyone, including partial prostheses for women who have had partial surgery, such as a lumpectomy. Advances are being made in this field all the time: for example, early prostheses tended to be quite heavy but now there are lightweight versions available. You can even get one that attaches painlessly to the chest wall so you don't need to wear a bra.

I'd been told I shouldn't wear a silicone prosthesis until six weeks after surgery but I couldn't wait that long and was keen to get one as soon as possible. I ended up waiting until Mum flew out to Australia and we went to Grace Bros together. It was about four weeks after my op and my scarring still looked quite vicious so I apologised in advance to the assistant as I didn't want my appearance to shock her. She was lovely and so kind, and not only did she kit me out with a prosthesis but also several new bras with full cups to accommodate it securely. They did have a range of mastectomy bras (which have a pocket concealed on the inside of the cup which the breast form slips neatly into), however I couldn't find any I really liked. I thought they were all a bit frumpy, so I just chose normal bras with large cups. Mum told me about a UK company, Nicola Jane, which sells mastectomy bras and swimwear. I love their bras because they are so pretty—very lacy and feminine—as well as extremely comfortable, and that makes you feel good—which is so important. Nicola Jane have a mail order catalogue and web site and deliver internationally. Amoena, an American company, also has pretty bras. So you don't have to look like you've borrowed one of your granny's bras! (For contact details see page 184.)

Now I had my breast back and I felt great!

In order to get full movement back into my left arm, I had to do various sets of exercises several times a day. There were about five different exercises, including putting your hands on your head and behind your back and standing next to a wall and crawling your fingers up it. Each time I would mark with a pencil how far up the wall I'd managed to stretch my fingers, wondering if I'd ever be able to extend my arm fully again. It still felt very tight—the exercises appeared to be so simple and yet were so difficult for me to do. However, I persevered and did my exercises religiously, determined that I would be able to use my left arm just as I had before the mastectomy. Ten days after coming out of hospital, I was driving.

Lymphoedema was also a concern for me. Lymphoedema is the retention of lymph (a liquid) in the tissues, resulting in swelling. It can occur when you've had any lymph nodes removed—removing lymph nodes is common in surgery for breast cancer, as you can tell from them whether the cancer has spread. These lymph nodes protect the arm from infection, so it becomes very important that you don't scratch, burn or cut your arm, as this could cause lymphoedema to develop. Stay out of the sun, no hot showers or baths, that kind of thing. Mum has lymphoedema in her left arm, and I know that that upsets her far more than having a mastectomy ever did. She wasn't warned about the possibility of it occurring, and shortly after her operation, did a bout of particularly vigorous cleaning and scrubbing. Her left arm swelled up and has never returned to its pre-op size. I'm left-handed so I can't not use my arm. In fact, I use it as I always did, but I just take extra care. Lymphoedema can be controlled in several ways, including specialised massage, wearing a compression sleeve and elevating the affected limb, all of which aid lymphatic drainage. Fortunately, I have been able to control the slight swelling I occasionally get with massage and without the need for a sleeve. Towards the end of my pregnancy my left arm became swollen but this disappeared following a massage after James' birth. The problem with lymphoedema is that it's not a condition that only affects you in the post-op period; the threat of it is with you for life.

Having a serious illness like cancer places extra demands on your body, and so diet and nutrition during this time is really important. A good diet will make you feel good, stronger in yourself—better able to cope with your treatment. You wouldn't go in to war on an empty stomach, and this could be the biggest battle you ever face in your life. There were many occasions when I simply didn't feel like eating, but I forced myself to, even if it was just something small. If you don't put fuel in your car, it'll eventually stop. If you don't put food inside your body, it'll just become weaker and weaker.

BLACKEST DAYS

One of the ways I found around my loss of appetite was drinking freshly squeezed juices and fruit smoothies or milkshakes. During the chemo, my mouth and gums became very sore—I got ulcers and cold sores and my gums bled terribly. I found it more beneficial to drink something cool and nutritious which was soothing to my mouth than to plough my way through a meal, which often made my mouth feel worse. People often talk about taking antioxidants in the fight against cancer and other diseases. One of the best ways to get these naturally is in freshly squeezed juices. Glenn and I already had a juicer so I went out and bought a book entitled *The Uses of Juices* which was packed with information and told me all about the health benefits to be found in different juices and juice combinations. It was only a small book but it was full of lots of juice recipes and combinations.

One of my favourites was orange and pineapple, which is absolutely delicious chilled. Every day I would drink at least one, preferably two, carrot, apple and beetroot juices—three carrots, two apples and one beetroot in each. The carrot and beetroot juice is especially good for building blood cells, so it was particularly beneficial during chemotherapy. Carrot juice contains twelve of the essential minerals for the human body. It is the richest source of vitamin A and also contains ample proportions of vitamins B1, B2 and C. It has strong antiseptic qualities, is an excellent blood cleanser and alkalinizer and as a bonus, it helps to clear and beautify the skin! Beetroot juice contains four vitamins and nine important minerals, and when it is combined with the carrot juice, it becomes one of the best natural builders of body cells. The not so humble apple contains nine of the sixteen chemical elements required by our bodies and four of the six important vitamins. It builds resistance to infection, is useful in changing colonic flora and reducing colonic bacilli, helps in the elimination of toxins, in the reduction of gallstones and is good for gout. It is also a good body cleanser, great for the complexion and good for loss of appetite. The benefits of fresh juices seem to be endless. As I drank, I would picture the power of the goodness from the juices circulating around my body—that made me feel great!

THE FIGHT GOES ON

I'd been out of hospital and at home for a week when I had my first appointment to go and meet Professor John Kearsley at St George Cancer Care Centre. He was to be in charge of my radiotherapy treatment. I was a little apprehensive, as I didn't really know what to expect, but luckily I had Glenn and my Mum along for moral support.

Radiotherapy, or radiation treatment, as it is sometimes known, uses rays such as x-rays, gamma rays or electrons to either cure or control the cancer. It works because the rays stop the cancer cells from growing. The rays can't differentiate between the cancer cells and the body's normal cells, but the cancer cells are unable to withstand the effects of the radiotherapy and die, whereas the normal cells recover, usually with no permanent damage. Radiotherapy is localised to a particular area, as opposed to chemotherapy, which affects all the cells in your body. There are two forms of radiotherapy treatment. Some people have radioactive implants put inside their body at the site of the cancer. These are small containers or wires filled with a radioactive substance. This is called internal radiotherapy. The other comes in the form of a machine like an x-ray machine, which directs rays specifically to the site of the cancer. You can't see the rays and neither can you feel them. This is known as external radiotherapy, and this is what I had.

We were shown into one of the radiotherapy rooms. It was fairly dark, but I could see beautifully painted murals over the ceiling—the reason for these was soon to become apparent. In the middle of the room was the kind of bed you'd see in a doctor's surgery, and right next to that a large x-ray machine. I lay down on the bed whilst the professor and radiotherapist marked out the precise area on my chest wall where the rays would be directed. This is known as the 'treatment field'. They then tattooed three tiny dots onto the area—they would use these to line the machine and rays up so that the radiotherapy was directed at the exact same spot each time I received treatment.

My course of radiotherapy was to last for five weeks, and would take about fifteen minutes per session. It was a two-week cycle. The first week I would go once a day for five days, the second week once a day for four days, and so on. On arriving at the centre, I'd take a seat and wait until my name was called. I then had to change into a long gown and go into the radiotherapy room. I would lie down on the bed and keep very still whilst the radiotherapists lined the machine up against the left side of my chest wall for my treatment. As well as having the dots, they would draw lines on the chest wall with a marker pen to help line the machine up. I discovered that this didn't easily come out of my undies when I dressed again after the treatment, so I allocated a couple of my bras as my radiotherapy bras. As you're lying down and looking up at the ceiling, you can look at the various murals while you're being zapped. There was also music playing,

THE FIGHT GOES ON

which helped to relax you if you were feeling a little tense. The radiotherapists operate the machine from a room next door so that they are not subjected to the effects of the rays, but they can still see you at all times, either through a window or on a television screen. The whole procedure takes just minutes and I found it totally painless.

My radiotherapy started in the middle of my chemotherapy, on 17 November, exactly two months after my mastectomy. Because the chemo runs for six months, the radiotherapy takes place within this time so that the ordeal is not prolonged even further. I chose to have my treatment at around 10 am, which meant we didn't have to be up too early but still had the rest of the day to enjoy. Glenn came to the Cancer Care Centre with me as often as he could, which was great. The staff and other patients always seemed to enjoy seeing him—it was nice to see people smiling there! I also made a friend there. I first noticed her because she was young too (the majority of patients were quite a bit older than myself), and I'd smile and nod. You're never quite sure if people want to talk at places like that but she smiled and nodded back, and we've been friends ever since. Her name is Sue, and she and her family lived not far from us in Cronulla. She'd also had breast cancer and had a lumpectomy, and like me, had been given a course of chemo and radiotherapy. We were often there at the same time, and when our names were called, we'd go and change into our gowns and sit and chat and laugh about how glamorous we looked until the radiotherapists were ready for us. It was a great distraction—you could almost forget why you were there!

The day after we'd been to meet Professor Kearsley, I had an appointment with a plastic surgeon to have a chat about reconstruction. It was a very positive meeting, although we wouldn't really be able to tell what route we'd take until we could see how my skin reacted to the radiotherapy treatment. I was optimistic that whatever the result, I would be able to have a reconstruction, which was fantastic news.

Two days later, I went with Mum to meet Dr Kiran Phadke, the oncologist in charge of my chemotherapy treatment, which was due to start the following week. He explained what would be happening and how long it would go on, and although I'd read about chemo, it was great to hear the facts first hand from an expert.

Chemotherapy is the use of drugs to kill cancer cells or slow down their growth. Cells grow by dividing. Chemotherapy works by damaging cancer cells that are dividing. The drug or drugs travel around the body in your bloodstream attacking cells—the cells which are most affected by chemo are those which divide rapidly. Chemotherapy attacks both cancerous and normal cells, but normal cells are able to renew themselves more quickly. Cancer cells recover more slowly and with more difficulty. The rest periods that you have in between your chemotherapy treatments are there to allow time for your normal cells to recover; the cancer cells do not recover, though, so more are killed with each treatment.

Chemotherapy can be given in different ways—by swallowing a tablet, as an injection to a vein or through a drip. My chemo was with tablets and injections. It began on Wednesday, 8 October, three weeks after my mastectomy. I had been absolutely dreading having to go for my chemo. I've never liked having injections. My legs turn to jelly and my heart beats nineteen to the dozen if I even so much as see a syringe. Just hearing the word chemotherapy filled me with fear. Glenn drove Mum and me down to Sutherland Hospital and we all caught the lift up to the fourth floor to the Oncology Room. I so did not want to be there. My feet felt like lead weights. I just wanted to run away back out to

THE FIGHT GOES ON

Wancobra, where I didn't have to deal with any of this. I was so frightened. Had Mum and Glenn not been with me, I don't know if I would have actually made it to the hospital.

The Oncology Room was much smaller than I had expected. It was a nice light room with a view across to the Sydney skyline in the distance. On the left-hand side there were about four or five beige vinyl recliner chairs, placed around the edge of the room, and on the other side there was a small office and a storeroom. When we first walked into the room, there were a couple of older people sitting in the recliners—they were hooked up to drips having their chemo administered by the nurse, who was dressed in a long gown and had gloves and a mask on. It was a sight that came as such a shock. My eyes welled up with tears and I was overcome by a wave of sheer disbelief and fear. I turned and ran out of the room and into the corridor, back to the lifts we'd just come up in.

Glenn came running after me and put his arms around me and held me. I cried that I simply could not go through with it. It was all just too much. Just when I thought I'd got through the worst bit, which I'd felt was actually agreeing to and having the mastectomy, the next hurdle presented itself, and it was far bigger than the last one. The nightmare had begun all over again. He held me tightly and whispered to me, 'I know this is hard for you, but the sooner you go in there and have the treatment, the sooner it'll all be over.' They were magic words. I knew that he was right, and that if I wanted to give myself the best possible chance at life, then I really didn't have a choice. I guess I just needed someone else to take control. I took a deep breath, wiped my tears away and we turned around and walked back to the Oncology Room together.

Mum was there waiting for us, chatting away to one of the

nurses. It must have been heartbreaking for her to see me in such a state and know there was nothing she could do. If she could, I know she'd have put herself in my place and had the chemo for me. The Oncology nurse came over and introduced herself to us as Michelle. She invited us to take a seat in the corner, which we did. She began explaining to us what would be happening, which drugs I was to be given and how their side effects might make me feel, including that my periods could stop and even the possibility of early menopause and infertility. The tears started flowing again—I just couldn't stop them. I felt overwhelmed by the whole experience. The reason she had to be covered with the gown, gloves and mask was because the chemo drugs are so toxic that she couldn't risk them accidentally getting on her in some way. They have to be toxic to kill any cancerous cells, but it was quite hard for me to take in that she couldn't risk getting any on herself and yet here was I having them actually injected into my bloodstream.

She asked which side I'd had the operation—this briefly cheered me up as it meant she couldn't tell which breast was the real one and which was the prosthesis. She gently inserted the needle into the back of my right hand; due to the risk of lymphoedema, it's advisable for me not to have any injections or blood pressure taken on my left arm. I was then hooked up to a drip. As the drugs entered my bloodstream, I felt a cool sensation run along the back of my hand. Before the actual chemo is injected, I was given a drug for nausea, as this is one of the most common side effects. The whole treatment took approximately twenty minutes, and it was all I could do to stop myself from ripping the needle out of the back of my hand and running out of the room. I began to feel extremely agitated, and desperate to get out of that room. I don't know how I actually remained seated there; it took every ounce of self-control I had. Mum put on a brave face throughout, when what she really wanted to do was sob her heart out. I guess she was just too close. She said recently that seeing me sitting there receiving my chemo just ripped her apart. She felt so helpless, but she had faith in the hospital staff and knew I was in good hands, which helped. She knew that Glenn was strong and that I was too.

By the time we had driven back to the flat, I felt as though I could physically have pulled my right arm off, the aggression was so great. I lay down and tried to rest but found it very difficult, as I was so worked up. I also started to feel nauseated—this continued until the Friday morning, by which time I began to feel much better. My next chemo injection was the following Wednesday, and as Glenn was away, Mum came with me again for support. I mentioned to Michelle, my nurse, how aggressive I had felt following the chemo last time, and she told me that it was a side effect of one of the drugs I had been given. She said she would discuss it with my oncologist and see if I could be given another drug in its place, which I was, thank goodness. I had decided to take a personal CD player with me, hoping that the music would distract me from what was actually happening and calm me down. Alas, it didn't work. I was just as tense.

My chemotherapy was in a four-week cycle. The first and second Wednesday of each month I would go to hospital for my injections. Before leaving Oncology after my first session, I was handed a little bottle of chemo tablets. I had to take three a day for two weeks. Michelle recommended that I take all three at night so that I would sleep through any side effects, which is what I did. It worked beautifully. With this cycle, my body had two weeks to recover and rebuild itself before the next onslaught the following month.

At one of my early chemo sessions, I met a man called

Graham, who was also there having his chemo. Michelle introduced us and I liked him immediately. He was young and had also been a flight attendant, and we'd sit and chat away about anything. Whenever I went in for my chemo, I always hoped that Graham would be there. He was so easy to talk to. Chatting away to him and Michelle made the chemo so much more bearable and the time flew by. I was thrilled when he and Michelle and their partners were able to come to our wedding.

As the weeks of chemotherapy passed, some side effects began to kick in. My eyes began to water uncontrollably, and I was forever dabbing at them with a tissue. Nothing I could do would make the watering stop. My left eye still waters from time to time. I felt and looked bloated, especially around my face. My mouth was an absolute mess. My lips became extremely dry and sore and I developed mouth ulcers that were painful and a nuisance. My gums were also sensitive, and would bleed often. My energy levels were very low—it became a real effort to do even the simplest things. The nausea was also ever-present. My hair thinned and came out in handfuls but I was very thankful that I didn't lose all of it. I had a selection of scarves and caps ready just in case.

At the beginning of each four-week cycle, I had to have a blood test to check that everything on the inside was okay. My first blood test after Christmas 1997 revealed that there was a problem with my liver. For some reason, it wasn't functioning properly. I panicked. It could mean a lot of things, including a secondary cancer, so I was utterly terrified. I was immediately booked into hospital for an abdominal CT scan. Luckily, Glenn was able to come with me, though he had a meeting later that morning which I insisted he kept. I was a nervous wreck that day, extremely anxious. Whilst we waited for my name to be called for my scan, I had to drink a bottle of vanilla-flavoured syrupy liquid (known as oral contrast) before I could have the scan. This just makes it easier for the radiographer to differentiate between the various organs and body tissue. As I sat drinking it, clutching Glenn's hand, a man on crutches approached Glenn, asking for an autograph and wanting a chat about cricket, completely oblivious to my presence and distress. Glenn signed for him, but I could not believe how anyone could be so selfish and insensitive. Surely there's a time and a place for things like that. Glenn had to leave for his meeting, and it was soon time for my scan.

I had to take off my clothes, change into a hospital gown and lie down on a cushioned bench around which the scanner would revolve. Before this I had to be injected with iodine, which would highlight my blood vessels. I was very tense and stressed about the whole situation and my reason for being there, and I hadn't realised I would have to have an IV. Once again, I had this feeling of utter disbelief at what was happening, and I fought back the tears as I lay there. The nurse was very kind and held my hand whilst the iodine was administered—I felt so childish, but I needed the comfort. I was left alone whilst the machine scanned my body—this takes a few minutes, during which time you have to keep very still. Afterwards, the iodine IV was removed and it was all over. I wanted to wait for the results. I couldn't leave the hospital without knowing, so after getting dressed I took a seat in the waiting room. It seemed to take forever before the same nurse came out to tell me that everything was fine—there were no problems with my liver or anything else. I was so relieved; the tears again welled up in my eyes, and this time they wouldn't stop flowing. Another hurdle successfully cleared.

During the final month of my chemotherapy, the side

effects seriously began to take their toll. I felt as though my whole body was falling apart. I was completely drained and run down, and developed a sore throat. My doctor prescribed antibiotics to treat it. This only succeeded in giving me a severe bout of thrush, just to add to my problems. To top it all, I also developed a thrombosis haemorrhoid. I didn't realise what the problem was at first as I'd never previously had one. I assumed I was just constipated, and sent Glenn out to the midnight chemist one night to buy me a magic cure to make me go to the toilet. I was so sore I couldn't sit down. I didn't know what to do with myself. Half of me was absolutely desperate to go to the toilet and the other half dreaded it because it felt as though I was passing broken glass and taking an eternity to do it. It was sheer agony. The pain was just awful. I wanted to go to the doctor but I felt terribly embarrassed. In the end, I could stand it no longer and took myself off to the surgery. I'd made an appointment with a lady doctor, and she was so kind. She told me I had a thrombosis haemorrhoid and that it was actually going away, thank heavens. I wished I'd been able to swallow my pride and had gone to see her sooner.

By this stage, I had reached the end of my tether. Everything was going wrong—it felt like one thing after another. My friend Sue from the radiotherapy sessions had told me that by the time she'd almost completed her chemo, she didn't think she could go through with her final injection. When she'd told me that, I hadn't been able to understand why she felt that way. I thought she'd be relieved that it was nearly all over at long last. Now I was nearly at the end of my chemo and I knew exactly how she felt. I'd had enough.

It was also during this time that Linda McCartney died from breast cancer. I was absolutely devasted by her death. She had stood for so many things that were good and true,

THE FIGHT GOES ON

and had been so brave and courageous in her fight. It was hard to believe that she'd gone.

I remember being determined that my life would not revolve around my chemo or change because of it. My friend Susan Porter, Mark Waugh's fiancée, was holding a clothes party the Wednesday afternoon of my second session of chemo and I had been adamant that I was going. Tracy was also going, and had driven over from Manly so that she could go with Mum and myself. I insisted on driving, even though I felt absolutely awful (I had also started my period the day before), but I didn't want to let Susan or Tracy down after I'd said I would be there. It was only a twenty-minute drive from our flat to Susan's. We were about two-thirds of the way there when I was hit by a wave of nausea and uncontrollable tears. I immediately pulled over and confessed to Mum and Tracy that I wasn't feeling too well but hadn't wanted to spoil their day, especially with Tracy having already travelled for an hour to get to our house. Tracy rang Susan from the car and gave our apologies; then drove Mum and me back to the flat, where I went straight to bed. Looking back, it seems silly that I even contemplated going out or socialising after a chemo session, but back then, I had been incredibly stubborn, and determined that it wasn't going to change my life. There were times when it had to, and I learned to live with that.

G I don't believe I will ever fully comprehend how badly the chemotherapy and radiotherapy knocked Jane about, because when Jane is happy, she's ecstatic, and when she isn't, she still puts on a smile and brave face and gets on with life. I wish I had her temperament on the cricket field—I have found myself in quite a bit of bother when I have let my frustrations get the better of me. Jane's a cool customer, and while the chemo and radiotherapy did drag her spirits down towards the end of her treatment—there was a time when she felt as if it was tearing her apart—she tried not to dwell too much on the negative side of her situation. And on the mornings when she couldn't drag herself out of bed she just said she needed rest; there were no hysterics or complaints. I used to just sit with her for hours at a time when she went to the hospital. Jane called me her 'rock', but I gained a lot more from her than she could have from me. Unlike chemo, doctors say that the administration of the radiotherapy is painless and similar to having an x-ray taken, but the process is dragged out because it takes a lot of time to get the patient into the right position, to ensure that they're given the right dosage of therapy and that it's applied to the right area. While the procedure *is* painless, the side effects, which take about a fortnight to surface, are less pleasant—they include fatigue, a loss of appetite, allergic-like skin reactions and bone marrow suppression. Jane suffered from a terrible itch, which drove her around the bend. I would watch in horror as she clawed at her affected skin . . . it was moist and red raw like the most severe sunburn, and as much as I hated doing it, I had to try and stop her from scratching herself because I knew it would only irritate her skin even more.

Towards the end of her treatment Jane loathed going to the hospital, and sometimes it became a battle of her will to enter the ward at Sutherland Hospital for treatment . . . the doctors struggled to give her the injections because the veins in her wrists and arms had started to close up. She loathed the chemo, and I well recall her feeling that she couldn't go on with it. Jane eventually summoned the courage and I couldn't help but feel proud when she marched back in and faced her fears— and pain—yet again. Sometimes she'd look bloated after the treatment, but unlike many other women Jane didn't lose much hair. She might have lost a handful at a time, but because she

THE FIGHT GOES ON

was so determined to hide the effects, I didn't really ever notice it ever looking too dramatic.

J My first goal following my operation was to get myself well enough to be able to travel up to Brisbane for the first Test of the 1997/98 Australian cricket season against New Zealand. When I set myself this goal, I had completely forgotten to take my chemotherapy into account, so I was extremely relieved when I realised the Test fell between injections. It was my second cycle of chemo. I had my injection on Wednesday, 5 November and flew up to Brisbane the following day, feeling a little worse for wear but determined to go. I even carted our juicer up with me so I could keep my vitamin intake up—I really felt the benefits. A few of the other wives and girlfriends were up in Brisbane too, so I knew that I wouldn't be by myself. It was my first 'public appearance' with the team since my operation and I desperately wanted to look exactly the same as I usually did, with not a care in the world. I didn't want to hide myself away under baggy clothes, so I just packed what I would normally take to Brisbane and hoped I'd be able to carry it off. I wanted Glenn to see that I was coping with everything—I wanted him to be proud of me. I also wanted to make sure that he was focused on the Test match and not worrying about me. The last thing I wanted was for my illness to affect his cricket and his career. I also felt it was important for the other girls to see that having breast cancer hadn't been the end of my world and that, on the surface at least, life hadn't changed at all.

I always look forward to the first Test in Brisbane. We stay at a beautiful hotel just across the road from the botanical gardens and it was really invigorating and a great start to the day to go for a brisk morning walk around them before heading off to the Gabba to watch a day's cricket. I love watching Glenn play. Anyway, we had a lovely few days up in Brisbane, won the Test and I flew home on Tuesday, 11 November ready for my next treatment on the Wednesday. My first goal, and I'd achieved it!

It was during this Test in Brisbane that Glenn first experienced trouble with a nerve entrapment, resulting in him being given the next two Tests off to enable him to have treatment on it. He actually went into hospital on 12 December to have the nerve killed as the problem wasn't getting any better and the cause of it remained a mystery. He then played in a one-day game in Adelaide where he suffered a slight strain to his stomach muscle. He wasn't too bothered by it, as the nerve had been killed previously. He went on to play in both the Melbourne and Sydney Tests against South Africa and it was during the Sydney Test that he ended up with a seven-centimetre long tear in his stomach muscle. He was out for the rest of the season, missing a tour to India and later on the Commonwealth Games. Despite it being very disappointing for Glenn, the up side of all of this was that he was able to be with me during what turned out to be the toughest months of my treatment. If he hadn't been injured I would have been left to cope without him.

My radiotherapy course of treatment finished on Tuesday, 23 December. Perfect timing! We caught the 1 pm flight from Sydney down to Melbourne, which is where the Test side spends Christmas in readiness for the Boxing Day Test—in 1997 it was against South Africa. We always end up taking so much luggage down to Melbourne—not only a bag crammed with the usual clothes and toiletries, but also bags of presents. This year was no exception. It's so exciting to get to Melbourne and see all the other wives and partners and their children. It's the only Test that everyone goes to. At this point, Michael Bevan wasn't in the Test side, which meant that he and Tracy weren't going to be down in Melbourne. I knew I would miss my best friend.

The area of my chest wall where the radiotherapy had been centred was by this time extremely sore, rather like a burn. I had dressings to put over it but the skin felt so tight. There was a chemist close to our hotel and I really wanted to go in there and explain my problem and see if he could prescribe a cream to soothe the area, but I was too embarrassed. In the end, the pain became so severe that I couldn't bear it, and Susan Porter talked me into going to the chemist. In fact, she practically frogmarched me down there! I took a deep breath and told him of my situation and he gave me a sorbolene cream that felt like cooling velvet on my red raw skin. I also began to get frequent, quite fierce shooting pains across my chest wall—at times they were so sharp they made me gasp and took my breath away. I'd been told this was the nerve endings in my chest and nothing to worry about, but knowing the cause didn't really help. Unfortunately, it was something I just had to put up with, as there was nothing I could take to make the pains go away. As the weeks passed, the intensity lessened, but it took approximately six months before they stopped altogether. On one day during the Test match, the pain was so bad and my skin so sore that I didn't go across to the MCG, which was unheard of for me. The girls were all brilliant, and rallied round, without making a fuss or feeling sorry for me. I couldn't have asked for more from my friends.

Throughout my chemotherapy and radiotherapy I was surrounded with the love and support of both old and new family and friends—something you simply cannot put a price on. It was so very important to me to know that I wasn't going through the nightmare alone. Tracy would send me beautiful cards filled with inspirational words when she knew I was struggling. I kept them all and I would read them again and again if I was having a bad day; they helped me to get through the really tough times. I also had my two beautiful cats—'the boys', as we called them—Simba and Tigger, and their presence helped me enormously too. I found it extremely comforting just having them around. It was all part of my support network. The one thing I couldn't do, and which I sometimes yearned for, was to be able to pick up a telephone and speak to someone who had been through exactly the same thing as me and who completely understood my thoughts and fears. I now know of at least one organisation that offers this kind of support to those of us whose lives have been affected by cancer. This is the Breast Cancer Support Service. (For details see page 183.) This kind of support is invaluable. Breast cancer, not just the mastectomy, but the chemo and radiotherapy that followed, was such an unknown entity. I wanted to be reassured that the way I was feeling was quite normal and that yes, in time, life would get back to normal and, as in my case, could be even better than ever.

G Jane and I decided early in the piece to keep her health problems out of the press. We'd been around long enough to realise that had her situation become public, there would have been numerous (and unwelcome) intrusions on our personal lives. I didn't want the media glare to distract Jane from the business of getting better, and I also wanted to be left alone to concentrate on playing cricket. I knew it was going to be a tough enough job to focus on getting wickets without the distraction of an army of journalists wanting to document her battle in the tabloids. In saying that, I must add that the journalists were tremendous. As you can imagine, the cricket world is a very small community, and it didn't take long for our sad news to leak out. Before long quite a number of pressmen were well aware that Jane had some serious problems. They realised it was a 'hot' story, and I think it is to their credit that upon hearing our request, they 'sat' on the story. While I have had one or two run-ins with some media guys over the years, I am very grateful that they respected our wishes—I have no doubt the privacy allowed us some much-needed room to breathe.

It's funny how destiny works: after my seven-wicket haul injury pretty well wiped me out of the rest of the 1997/98 season. The trapped nerve made life very bloody difficult. I couldn't stretch, and sometimes when I did something as simple as get out of bed in the morning or even sneeze it felt as if a sharp knife had been stabbed deep into my groin. And attempting to bowl at 140-odd kilometres an hour was painful, to say the least.

The pain wouldn't cease, and the Australian Cricket Board arranged for me to visit one of the nation's top neurosurgeons so he could try to deaden the 'rogue' nerve with high frequency treatment. It was a bit like a medical version of pin the tail on the donkey, and it took the doctor three attempts before he finally hit the right spot. My rehabilitation took a lot longer than I wanted it to, and I missed the final two Tests against the New Zealanders. I'd be lying through my teeth if I said it wasn't a frustrating time. The surgeon suggested I undergo a pain management course. The irony of the situation wasn't lost on me when I thought of Jane and the other cancer patients I'd met during the course of her treatment, who are left to fend for themselves. Since I was an injured athlete with a profile, I had doctors all over me, and reports of my progress were tabled in the media with all the urgency of an important political or diplomatic matter. I know sport makes news and that news helps to make the world go round, but it was hard to make sense of the attention when I was at home and alone with my girlfriend, who had fought the mother of all battles in silence. While she was being hammered from pillar to post by the awful side-effects of her treatment, I had surgeons making appointments for me to learn all about pain management. Sure, I was grateful, but it didn't add up.

While I was in pain—and with a capital 'P'—I was still bitterly disappointed at being ruled out against the Kiwis, because I was confident it would take me a few steps closer to my ultimate career goal—being Test cricket's greatest-ever wicket-taker. Missing out made it hard to relax at home. Indeed, I'm afraid there were times when I expressed my frustration to poor Jane. I didn't handle the set-back too well. Despite her own problems, Jane was extremely supportive, and sometimes when I heard her talk and offer me her encouraging comments I had to stop and remind myself; 'Hang on mate, she's been fighting cancer.' In my defence, I must say that my cricket is as important to Jane as it is to me. Indeed, before the first ball of the Test series was even bowled, Jane made it clear that her goal was to be well enough to follow the circuit around Australia. The player's wives and partners are a close-knit group, and there are some firm friendships among them. They really come into their own when we're on tour, and the girls support one another. When Jane's battle with breast cancer became public knowledge, most of the player's partners not only phoned or visited us, but they also went en masse for check-ups at their nearest breast cancer clinic. While some of them discovered lumps, we were happy to hear that no one had anything to worry about.

And if Jane's goal was to be well enough to follow the cricket circuit I had no doubt she'd be well enough. Jane's a winner. I like her philosophy towards cricket and winning . . . she reckons if it takes sledging, bouncers or full-on aggro to keep Australia's winning record in the black, then it has to be done. With that type of support behind me I made a premature return for a one day international match in Adelaide—it was another poor decision, because I ended up with a post-hernia nerve problem. On top of my groin and a slight stomach injury, it meant I was stuffed.

As frustrating as it was, when I look back over that period of my life, it was almost as if destiny allowed me to stay home with Jane. I am grateful that the decision to stay at home was made for me by things outside of my control—I'm glad I didn't need to decide between staying in Sydney with Jane or playing for Australia. It might sound harsh, but professionally there was a lot on the line and Jane was adamant from the outset that her illness should not affect the way we lived our lives. And she made it very clear that my playing gave her something to focus on outside her illness.

In all honesty I wanted to play. Since Jane's health problems became public knowledge I have been asked on numerous occasions whether or not I took any of my frustrations out on batsmen, and the answer is a resounding no. Cricket was an escape for Jane as a spectator and me as a player, but had I surrendered to my emotions and bowled short at the batsmen or even bruised them it wouldn't have achieved anything for the team or Jane. If a doctor had said I could help Jane fight the cancer by branding the batsmen with a bouncer, I'd have gone on a six stitcher safari, but the truth about cricket is that you have to try and stay in control at all times.

Jane and I went down to Melbourne when it was thought I could force my way into the team which played South Africa in the Boxing Day Test. To do that I had to undergo a fitness test. It was some test, too. The ACB arranged for me to take part in a 'phantom' Test at Melbourne's Old Collegian ground for the two days leading up to the match. My challenge started at 11 am, when I was bowling to a Melbourne first grade batsman Chris Matthews who the Cricket Board had hired for the day. The journalists covering my quest enjoyed a bird's eye view since most of them served as fieldsmen. It was a real slog to motor through this, because as much as I hated to admit it, I was operating on only two cylinders. When the crunch came I couldn't give the selectors my word that I could bowl 20 overs a day at express pace, but they still picked me. I finished with match figures of 2-77 from 45 overs and while they were far from my best I was pleased with them under the circumstances.

When the selectors said they were going to leave the decision about my playing South Africa in the New Year's Day Test in Sydney to me, I think they knew there was no way on earth I was going to say no. At that stage I would have crawled over broken glass to retain the right to wear my Baggy Green—and the pain in my abdominal muscles was so bad I almost had to crawl.

There were some doubts about my ability to last the five-day Test match, however, I made a vow to myself that if I played then I would complete the match, no matter how hard that proved to be. Thankfully the first seven overs were fine and I dismissed my chosen match nemesis Gary Kirsten before my injury flared up in the eighth over. I allowed for myself to feel good, and bloody well jinxed myself. I made the mistake of relaxing, and ended up with a seven-centimetre tear in my abdominal muscles. It hurt like hell. I left the field for emergency treatment and Errol Alcott taped the area up in an attempt to help hold everything in place. It still hurt but I returned to the field and because of my pre-Test vow to finish the match no matter what, I didn't dare complain. While I usually like to switch off from the other parts of my life once I walk through the gates to play, I couldn't help but think of

THE FIGHT GOES ON

Jane's courage when I was finding the going tough. She was in the crowd with the girls, and I wanted to let her know that I could dig deep when I had to.

J I was due to have my final injection of chemotherapy on 29 April 1998, and I wanted it to be a celebration. I knew that Graham also would be there having his chemo, so I decided to bake a batch of chocolate chip cookies, enough for everyone. It was my way of saying a little thank you for helping to make my chemo sessions bearable. Glenn came in with me and we walked into the Oncology Room with smiles all over our faces—at last, we'd reached the end! I was so happy that it was all about to be over. I gave Michelle the cookies, took my seat, and our usual routine began. As she'd had a bit of trouble finding a vein on the last couple of occasions, I was prepared this time, and had put an anaesthetic patch over what I considered to be a particularly large vein in my foot. If worst comes to worst, I thought, I can have my injection down there.

Unfortunately for me, the worst did come to the worst. Michelle could not find a vein anywhere on my right hand, wrist or arm, and believe me, she did her best to find one. My veins just kept collapsing. I tried to remain positive; this was my last injection, after all. I told her I had stuck an anaesthetic patch on my foot and invited her to try that vein. The situation was beginning to look a little desperate, so she decided to take a look at the vein, which appeared quite promising. I was sure that this vein would work. Several attempts later, Michelle still had no joy. The problem was that my veins had basically had enough of the prodding and piercing over the previous six months and now, as soon as a needle was inserted into them, they constricted, thus preventing any blood flow.

By this stage, I was extremely upset. I was fighting back tears—I didn't want the others to see my distress. I didn't want anyone to feel sorry for me. I never have done and never will—it's such a waste of emotion and just makes you feel even worse. Glenn was by my side, doing his best to comfort me but I was beyond anyone being able to make it better. All I wanted him to do was hold my hand, which he did. I had entered that room with the biggest smile on my face, knowing it was my final session. Now everything was going horribly wrong, and here I was crying my heart out in front of everyone. I had thought that I'd got through the worst, but I had been wrong about that too. I felt embarrassed about baking cookies for everyone, and disappointed in myself for allowing my smile to be replaced by tears. I felt ashamed of myself for losing control and I knew I had to somehow pull myself together and deal with this situation. I had to have my chemo, there was no way I could get out of it. I asked Michelle if I could leave the room and have some time by myself to get my act together. I raced to the Ladies and sat in there alone and sobbed and sobbed. What were we going to do?

After a few minutes, Michelle came to find me. She gave me a big hug. She said she'd called a doctor, explained our situation and he was now on his way down to help out. I wiped the tears from my cheeks, took a big deep breath and walked back to the room with her and took my seat in between Graham and Glenn, apologising for my tears and trying to make light of the situation as best I could without actually meeting anyone's eyes. The doctor was very kind, and explained that he felt our best option was to insert a canula into the back of my right hand and administer the chemotherapy through that. He said he'd pop a little anaesthetic into the back of my hand first, as the procedure might be a

THE FIGHT GOES ON

bit painful. He advised me not to look, as the needle was quite large. That was all I needed to hear, and I immediately averted my gaze. Much to my amazement, I noticed Glenn sat there and watched the whole thing! The next thing I heard was Michelle saying that it had worked—the blood was flowing and so was the chemotherapy. This time the tears were of relief—finally, it was all over and ok. Things hadn't exactly gone according to plan, but the end result was the same, and after about twenty-five minutes, Glenn and I finally said our good-byes and walked out of that room and left the fourth floor for the last time. It was one of the best feelings in the world.

It was my birthday a few days later. I was thirty-two and we celebrated by moving into our beautiful new home. It has a deepwater frontage and backs onto the Royal National Park. It was a completely new start for us, and I felt as if I'd been born again. You know, it really is quite amazing how much we all take for granted in our lives, particularly the simple things in life, like waking up every morning and feeling well. Before I had cancer, I never even thought about feeling well and healthy or being able to do the most basic but necessary things in life, like going to the toilet, eating and sleeping. They're just things we do every day, week in week out, month in month out, year in year out, without once thinking how lucky we are to be able to live like that.

Now I am so very grateful to wake up in the morning and feel well. I celebrate these supposedly 'simple' things in my life and thank God for them every day. We rarely appreciate just what we have until it's taken away. Every day is a bonus, and if it's filled with blue skies and sunshine, then so much the better! On top of that, to be able to share it with someone who makes your heart sing and whom you love with every inch of your soul is almost indescribable. I can't believe how fortunate I am, and I have to be honest and say that if I hadn't had breast cancer, I doubt that my life would be as rich and fulfilling as it is now. I wouldn't change a thing, not a single moment, if I am who I am today because of having had cancer.

When I look back now and think about some of the things that used to be important to me or that I'd worry about before I was ill, I can't believe I wasted so much of my precious time in such meaningless pursuits. Glenn and I were now living in a house with the most beautiful view where kookaburras would fly in every afternoon at 4 o'clock to be hand-fed a piece of frankfurt, and the rainbow lorikeets, crimson rosellas and many other parrots come to feed. Our beautiful cats, Simba and Tigger, were my constant companions, always at my side and a source of much amusement. We had found out truly who our real friends were—those people who supported us and stood by us through what was an extremely traumatic time for everyone. They weren't afraid to call to see how we were going or if they could help us in any way. They didn't worry about saying 'the right thing' or 'the wrong thing', or cross the road if they saw us coming. They were simply themselves and were there for us in every way and we thank them for that from the bottom of our hearts.

Part Three

HAPPY EVER AFTER

ON TOP OF
THE WORLD

J With the course of chemo completed, I then had to go for three-monthly check-ups with Professor Kearsley at St George Cancer Care Centre. I was extremely nervous before my first check-up. I dreaded hearing him tell me that he'd found another lump or that I had a secondary elsewhere. For those first few months after surgery, there was this awful voice at the back of my mind saying, *What if it comes back, what if it comes back?* I was angry with myself for allowing this negative thought to enter my head and fought it whenever it did. I discussed my fears with Professor Kearsley and he assured me they were only natural given what I'd just been through. Of course there was a possibility that either of the situations I dreaded could happen, but he promised me that if they did, we'd treat them and beat them, just as we had this time. I left my first check-up with a clean bill of health and felt like I'd won the lottery! I walked out of the centre floating on air and still feel that way after every check-up, which are now six-monthly.

I don't think my life will ever get back to 'normal' again,

and nor would I want it to. I've been given a second chance and I intend to make every day count.

Whenever Glenn goes away on an overseas tour, our phone bills are always sky high. We like to talk on the phone at least once every day, sometimes more, depending on what's happened in the match or if something's happened at home. On one occasion whilst on a tour of Pakistan during October 1998, we were having our usual daily chat and got on to the subject of the upcoming Test Series against England in Australia. I always aim to go to as many of the Australian Tests as possible—if I didn't, I'd hardly get to see Glenn! We were discussing which Tests I would go to and I said I'd like to go to all of them with the exception of Perth, simply because the flight was a little longer and I knew that not many of the other girls would be going to that game. Glenn seemed surprised that I'd want to leave Perth out, and reminded me that it was where I flew out to first watch him play in a Test match against the Sri Lankans back in December 1995, and that we had some great memories there. He wanted me to go, and as it was obviously quite important to him, I happily agreed to use up some more of our frequent flyer points and go to Perth as well. Little did I know that he had special plans for us there.

The Perth Test was to start on the Friday. The evening before the Test, 26 November, there was to be a black tie dinner in honour of both teams. The year before I had been caught out when I didn't have anything suitable to wear for the dinner—Tracy Bevan and I had to borrow clothes from Judi Taylor. This year I was better prepared, and was in the lengthy process of getting ready when Glenn returned to the hotel room after a training session.

I was sitting at a table near to the window painting my nails when he walked in, gave me a kiss and plonked himself down on the bed. Nothing unusual there. He beckoned me to join him and I explained that I was in the middle of doing my nails and couldn't, and besides that, he was a bit smelly after training. I eventually gave in and went and lay down next to him. We were chatting away when out of the blue, he announced that he'd got me a present. He'd had to go into town earlier in the day and he'd bought me something. I love getting presents (who doesn't) and Glenn told me to close my eyes and hold out my hands while he fetched it. I was quite excited, but had no idea about what he might have bought for me. I was hoping for a box of chocolates. He quickly returned and sat down on the bed in front of me. He told me he loved me and then I felt him place a small box into my cupped hands. He told me I could now open my eyes.

When I saw the little box my heart skipped a beat and my eyes began to fill. Glenn slowly opened the box for me and inside sat the most beautiful sparkling white diamond solitaire engagement ring! I could not believe my eyes! When he asked me to be his wife, I wasn't able to answer straight away—the tears came first. Part of me just couldn't believe he was actually asking me to marry him. Deep down I knew that he was being serious, but part of me thought he was pulling my leg. I don't know why I thought he'd joke about something like that—I think I was in shock. When I realised he definitely meant it, I just screamed, I was so happy. I'm sure the whole hotel must have heard me. I hugged him so hard, I couldn't let him go. I think I said 'yes' about ten times. I just couldn't believe it—it was such a huge shock but such a fantastic surprise. He placed the gorgeous ring on my finger—it looked absolutely stunning.

I asked him how he'd managed to arrange everything without my knowing and he explained. I couldn't believe he'd managed to do all that and keep it a secret from me. The reason he'd proposed now, before the game, was because he wanted me to wear the ring at the Test match dinner that evening for everyone to see. He probably wanted it out of the way so he could focus on the match, too. You have to get your priorities right, after all!

G Jane wanted to get married and she wanted the whole shebang; a white dress...church...all our family and friends...fine food and litres of good drink...music and dancing...pageboys and flower-girls. I took my time in getting hitched and sometimes—just to torment her—I would talk about marriage and how special it must for two people to say 'I do'. Then, in the same breath, I would quickly change the subject and talk about the weather or the crowd we'd played in front of at our last match. Each time I spun my yarn I would watch Jane's eyes widen in the anticipation of me asking the BIG question but the words she so dearly wanted to hear never left my mouth. Ultimately, Jane grew tired of what she called my schoolboy-type 'gee-ups' and ordered me to stop dangling the carrot before her nose because she was sick and tired of the false hope. After a while, I was told not to even utter the word marriage unless I was deadly serious about doing something. Eventually I was ready for it. When I was on tour in Pakistan, sitting in a hotel room in Karachi, it just dawned on me that it was time for Jane and me to get married. It made sense because we'd always been comfortable together—even that first time when she arrived in Perth to see me despite wondering what the heck she was doing. In time, and it really wasn't all that long, we both realised we were true soulmates and the depth of our love was tested on a few occasions—my cricketing commitments and Jane's illness. In the time we have known each other Jane and I have climbed many mountains together, one much higher than any other, but when we came to the toughest part of the climb we held hands and conquered it.

Jane was everything I'd imagined in my future wife when I was an aspiring Test cricketer living alone in a caravan park picturing what I wanted my 'dream' life to be like. She has tremendous attributes including loyalty, courage, humour and compassion and she helped to build a real home for the pair of us with her personal touches around the unit. Sometimes it embarrasses Jane to tell people we met in a Hong Kong dive like Joe Bananas. In Jane's ideal world our eyes would have locked for the first time at a more romantic location such as on top of the Eiffel Tower in Paris or in an art gallery in Rome. I have no such regrets—I'm just grateful our paths crossed. I have no doubt our meeting was destiny and I sometimes wonder what my life would now be like had Brendon Julian not summoned the courage to approach the flight crew and announce that a few Aussie cricketers wanted to not only meet them but to share a drink or two. I think I can say in all confidence that without Jane, my life would not have been anywhere near as fulfilling as it has been, despite what has so far been a successful enough cricket career. Indeed, while I'm no Tom Cruise I could relate to the Hollywood film star when he won the Golden Globe award for *Magnolia*. Cruise said of his wife, actress Nicole Kidman, 'Her generosity, her support, her sacrifices, her talent—she inspires me.' I can understand where Cruise's words came from because Jane has helped me to be a better man. Indeed, it was with those kind of thoughts whirling around in my head at a million miles an hour in downtown Karachi that I decided it was time to put a ring on her finger.

I wanted to make the actual proposal something Jane would long remember, so I sought out the advice of our friend Tracy Bevan. If anyone could help me bowl the maiden Steele over, I knew it would be Tracy. She was sworn to secrecy, and I'm sure keeping mum must have made her want to burst because Tracy and Jane are so close. Tracy told me where she'd bought her diamond and I did the rest.

I knew the engagement ring I wanted for Jane . . . I could see it in my mind before I even started searching for it . . . and I found it for real in a Sydney jewellers when my manager, and good mate Warren Craig and I were amid a round of important appointments. We were there to finalise a radio deal and also to fine tune my cricket contract with the Australian Cricket Board and I'm very glad Warren was on hand to deal with the business side of things, because my mind was on the ring. As luck would have it, I found the stone I wanted after just a few hours. It was perfect, but I was presented with a problem of sorts when the jeweller said he couldn't have it ready in time for the date I intended to propose—on the eve of the Second Test in Perth. When I explained my predicament, the jeweller drew plans and made arrangements for a colleague in Perth to set the diamond in time.

I decided to propose to Jane at the Hyatt in Perth because I still view the hotel as a symbolic place for us. It was where Jane met me after she decided to take a punt and see whether an Aussie she met in a Hong Kong bar was worth worrying about. Being a romantic at heart I tried to get the same room we had stayed in that very first time, but it had already been booked. However, I refused to let that little hiccup spoil the moment. I rehearsed my lines a couple of dozen times. It was late in the afternoon before I summoned the courage to say what I wanted to.

Jane was busy getting ready for the team dinner—doing her

nails—when I asked her to join me on the bed (I figured it would be the softest place for her to land in case she fainted) because I had something to give her—and this time it wasn't five days' worth of cricket tickets! Jane told me to wait until she finished her nails, but I knew I had to seize the moment, and I insisted she put the nail polish down. I wanted to make my proposal memorable, so I told her how happy I was and how far I thought we had come since that fateful night in Hong Kong; I said how I'd admired her courage in fighting the breast cancer and how I figured it had made us a lot closer; I said the ordeal had not only proved we could confront anything life dealt us head-on but also proved she was the person I wanted to spend the rest of my life with. After that softening up period I went for the knockout, and asked Jane to close her eyes because I had something special for her. When I was certain she wasn't peeking, I said: 'I would be very proud if you would be my wife. Will you marry me?' Well, Jane got a bit emotional ... she screamed, and I mean screeeee-amed! In hindsight, it was just as well I didn't ask for her hand in marriage at a restaurant or some other public place—who knows what people may have thought? Then Jane burst into tears. Once she realised she hadn't given me an answer, she squealed 'Yes, yes, yes and yes!' It was brilliant and just to let her know it wasn't another joke I said to her; 'You always gave me a hard time for dangling that carrot before you, well, put one on your finger!' The ring fit perfectly, just like us.

We had some champagne and I celebrated by having a massage to help prepare myself for the Test. Well, Jane can't keep a secret and it didn't take long for the boys to hear of our happy news.

J I think the first person I called was Tracy. She'd known about Glenn's plans all along and hadn't given even so much as a hint. Though I did think it was strange one Sunday morning when I'd popped out to get the newspapers and come back to see Glenn standing in the office wearing not much more than a smile, chatting away to Tracy on the phone. She'd called and started leaving a message on our answering machine and he'd leapt out of bed and raced into the office to grab the call before she hung up. He made up some story about her ringing to get some information for Michael and said that she didn't need to talk to me, which was a first. I didn't really believe him, but I couldn't imagine what else he'd be covering up so I let it go.

When I rang to tell her that Glenn had proposed, she was almost as excited as I'd been. After about fifteen minutes of screaming and crying on the phone to her, I thought I'd better give my parents a call and let them know. They were absolutely thrilled to bits, as were Glenn's family. Glenn had to go off for a team meeting before the dinner, so I decided to give Kelly Sainty, Ricky Ponting's then girlfriend, and Lindsay Campbell, Michael Kasprowicz's fiancée, a call on the pretext of helping me get ready for that evening. Kel was round first. She'd had a nasty eye infection and was thinking about not going to the dinner. I had to talk her out of that! She was pretty down, saying she didn't think she could go. I stood in front of her with my left hand on my chin, waggling the third finger, wondering how long it would be before she noticed. It seemed to take forever—maybe it was her dodgy eye—but eventually she saw it and screamed. It was the reaction I wanted. Lins arrived soon after and I told her I couldn't decide whether I liked my nail varnish and what did she think, placing my left hand under her nose. More screams, and then some champagne from room service.

When we went down to dinner, I couldn't wipe the smile or the glow from my face. Word of our engagement quickly began to spread. The girls and other dinner guests were shown to our tables and both our boys and the England team were taken backstage whilst everyone else took their seats. When the audience was seated, the boys came on stage and were individually introduced by the MC, then they sat down at their respective tables. Ricky Ponting was one of the first boys out and before sitting down he came over to congratulate me and planted a kiss on my cheek, bless him. A couple of the others followed suit—I was the most popular girl in the room! When the formal proceedings were over, Glenn and I rounded the evening off by sharing a bottle of Dom Perignon in the bar with the Pontings and the Kaspers—the perfect end to a perfect day.

The amount of cricket the boys play these days is enormous. I think Glenn had originally fancied a long engagement, but when we sat down and began to work out possible dates for our wedding, it was either July 1999 or April 2002! I'm sure he'd have been happy with 2002 but I had other ideas, and we set the date for 17 July 1999. Glenn would be overseas from February until late June with the tour of the West Indies and then the World Cup in England. I was due to join him in Barbados mid-April, so the wedding was organised fairly quickly.

I left to join Glenn in Barbados on 21 April. Susan Porter and I had decided to travel together to Barbados via London, where we would pick up Tracy Bevan. The Sunday before we left I'd popped over to Sue's for an hour and returned home to be greeted by my neighbour who told me that our little black cat, Tigger, had been run over and killed just at the front of our house. I was absolutely devastated and just could not believe that such a thing could have happened—we live in such a quiet street. Thankfully, they'd picked Tigger up for me and wrapped him up. He looked as though he was just sleeping. I rang Sue in hysterics and she came straight over, as did our friends Pam and Greg Lee, who buried Tigger in the garden for me. I was absolutely heartbroken. The following morning, Greg came round with a little coffin he'd made for Tigger and we put him in that, re-burying him in his favourite part of the garden with lots of lizards and birds around. I was so upset I almost cancelled my trip to Barbados. Glenn talked me back into going—I was desperate to see him too.

The boys had been away on a tour of the West Indies since mid-February. Whenever they're away on tour, the newspapers are full of photographs of what the boys get up to whilst they're overseas. I nearly died one day when I opened the paper to see a photo of Glenn and Steve Waugh standing right on the edge of a ledge at Kaieteur Falls in Guyana. On another occasion, while touring South Africa, Glenn called, telling me he was depressed, fed up and missing me. By the time the call was over, I felt depressed myself. I went and made a cup of tea and switched on the early evening news. I was just in time to catch the sports report and footage of the Test team in South Africa. I could not believe my eyes when they showed footage of Glenn hurtling down a water slide at Sun City in a little pair of Speedos, grinning from ear to ear and apparently having the time of his life!

The girls had all been looking forward to a well-deserved week in Barbados. Shopping for a bikini had proved a little awkward for me but I was determined to wear one with pride and not hide myself away under a billowing shirt. I eventually bought a couple of bikinis with little cropped tops, which were perfect.

The boys were there to meet us at the airport and we

travelled with them by bus back to the apartments they were staying at. There was one more one-day game to go before the tour was over. We all went to it. After that game, we all moved to a hotel right on the beach and stayed there for a week. It was great to be able to relax for a few days without the pressure of a game looming.

One day we all went out on a yacht for the day, cruising the azure waters of the Carribbean. At lunchtime we moored off a gorgeous little beach with turtles swimming nearby. It was a hot day and the clear water looked so inviting that before long everyone was in the water and I was the only one left on the yacht. I felt a bit left out; I so wanted to take a dip but was worried about my prosthesis falling out and either sinking to the bottom of the sea or floating on the surface. I was filled with horror at either prospect. Tracy had been for a swim and came back on board so I told her my problem. She said she'd come with me and stay close, and if anything popped out, she'd quickly grab it. Oh, what the heck, I thought, and decided to give it a whirl. I started to climb down the steps into the warm water. Treading water close by was Geoff Marsh (then the Australian coach). He'd been snorkelling and was now ready to come aboard for lunch. I seized my opportunity. 'Don't take your snorkel off just yet, Geoff,' I told him. 'You might be required to make a quick dive to the bottom at any second!' We were all laughing so much he couldn't have climbed aboard if he'd tried. And he did wait for me to have my swim—which was extremely refreshing and incident-free—before he got out of the water, bless him.

After a week of relaxing in the Barbados sunshine and topping up the tan, it was time to head for England and the World Cup. I was looking forward to the World Cup, partly because it gave me an opportunity to catch up with my family and friends, many of whom hadn't seen me since the last Ashes tour in 1997, when I first discovered the lump in my breast.

Each team participating in the World Cup had a base, and the Australian team was allocated Cardiff, in Wales. On the previous Ashes tour, we had been allowed to stay with the boys during the Tests but not during the games in between. We had quickly discovered that wherever the team was due to play, all of the accommodation in that town had been booked out well beforehand, making it extremely difficult for us to find somewhere to sleep. For this World Cup we were allowed to stay with the boys, so we didn't have to find our own accommodation, thank heavens. We all had cars to get around in. Susan and I shared one—I was the driver and she was the navigator. We made a great team, bombing up and down the motorways of Great Britain.

There were a couple of warm-up matches before the start of the World Cup. Our first World Cup match was against Scotland in Worcester on 16 May. We won that, then it was back to Cardiff for our next match, against New Zealand. Next was Pakistan at Headingley (Leeds) all in the space of about a week. It was during this time that I realised I was supposed to be having my period, but nothing had happened. I didn't think about it too much, sure that it would occur sooner or later. After the Pakistan match on the Sunday, the boys were travelling further up north to Durham so I decided to go down to Norfolk and spend some time with my Mum instead. Mum and I did the usual girly things—cream cakes, Banoffee pie, shopping, etc—and it was whilst I was with her for a few days that I began to get an inkling that I actually might be pregnant. I didn't want to get too excited. After all, I had been warned several times that the chemotherapy could make me infertile, though it hadn't stopped my periods as they said it might. I didn't say much to Mum though she did begin to wonder why I was going to the loo all the time. I think she suspected.

I was desperate to do a pregnancy test but I didn't want to do it without Glenn being there. I was due to drive up to Manchester to stay with him that Friday so I bought a couple of tests to do as soon as I got there. Norfolk is in the southeast of England and Manchester is in the north, so it was a fair journey. It ended up taking me just over four hours to drive from Mum's to Manchester and by the time I reached the boys' hotel, I was absolutely desperate to go to the loo. I dashed up to Glenn's room and hammered on the door. When he opened it, I gave him a quick kiss hello and disappeared into the bathroom with the pregnancy test hidden in my pocket. Very excited and very nervous, I did the test and waited. I was both shocked and overjoyed to see the blue lines appear almost straight away to tell me that, yes, we were having a baby. I wrapped the wand in a flannel and casually walked out of the bathroom and over to Glenn who was lying on the bed talking on the telephone.

I was bursting to tell him the news and stood in front of him, frantically making signals to him to wrap up the call and get off the phone. When he eventually did, I unfolded the flannel and presented him with the pregnancy wand. He didn't understand what was going on until I told him that we were having a baby. He was totally floored. I don't think he could actually believe it. For some reason, he thought I was joking—I guess it was the shock.

I wanted to tell Tracy straight away as I'd already told her my period was late. I gave her a call and invited her up for a cup of tea. I think she was on her way before I'd finished talking. She came up quickly, followed by Michael, and we told them our brilliant news. I think Trace was as happy as

I was—we hugged and cried while the boys stood there thinking we'd gone completely mad.

The next day, 30 May, the boys had a 'must win' game against the West Indies at Old Trafford and Glenn went out and took 5–14 in 8.4 overs. Australia went on to win the match and qualify for the Super Sixes. I'd like to think that was Glenn's way of showing he was pretty pleased about my news!

One of the highlights of the World Cup, apart from actually winning it, was being invited up into the boys' dressing room at Lord's after the presentations. After the game, everyone walked out onto the ground to watch the presentation on the balcony. After the boys had been given the Cup and their winners' medals, Glenn and a few of the others came down to us with hugs and champagne. It was brilliant to be able to share the moment. Shortly after, someone came to fetch us to take us up into the dressing room. We thought that there must be some mistake. Women simply aren't allowed in the Lord's Pavilion, let alone inside the dressing room. But it was true and up we went. There were a few raised eyebrows as we walked up the stairs, giggling and chattering away excitedly, but we were absolutely thrilled to bits. In the dressing room, the atmosphere was amazing, and it was so great to be a part of it. We had a drink with the boys and held the Cup and then left them to it. It was a very special experience and one I shall never forget.

If I had any complaints about being a player's wife on that World Cup tour it would have to be about the seating arrangements made for us at the respective grounds. Why do they always have to seat us with family and friends of the opposition? All I can say is, it's a good job I wasn't born a man, because I'd be in so many fights and scrapes it wouldn't be funny. Fortunately Tracy Bevan is exactly the same. Actually, she's probably worse than me. It must be the English. We'd sit together at the games and it would never be long before some bright spark would decide to dish out some armchair advice to one of our husbands or call him something unrepeatable. It makes you laugh because more often than not, you'll turn round, only to see some big fat blob who's never achieved anything in his life but after a few beers thinks he's got the right to abuse someone who has. I simply cannot sit there and listen to that without giving out a bit of advice of my own, and I can guarantee it would happen at every game. If you think it's aggressive on the field, you should sit in the stands next to Tracy and me!

Even though it was great to be back in England and catch up with everyone for those few weeks during the World Cup, I just couldn't wait to get back to Sydney, and Simba. I feel as though I've always lived here—it's home now. There was also a wedding to organise.

G Jane and I wanted to start a family, but we figured that could take years—and we feared it would also take more than a sprinkling of luck to enjoy the miracle of life so many couples take for granted. The surgeon's warning that the chemotherapy treatment could well leave Jane infertile was certainly on our minds, but we still decided to try—and hope. So when she told me in that Manchester hotel room that she was pregnant I was thrilled. Her words took a second or two to register but the funny thing is that just a few days before her test I had a nagging suspicion she was pregnant. Call it a fast bowler's intuition, if you will, but when she told me the news it didn't come as so much of a shock to me. I think my initial reaction might have disappointed Jane—I didn't scream the place down and look for a bottle of champagne to crack open—but I swear

I was chuffed ... really chuffed ... to think I was going to become a father. Me, a dad!

Everyone was thrilled for us, but even though I was so happy at the thought of becoming a father, I didn't fully appreciate what it meant until we returned to Australia and I saw an ultrasound of our baby. I could see this tiny heart beat-beat-beating. The meaning of it struck me like a bolt of lightning and I felt teary-eyed.

While we were in England I finalised a deal with the Worcestershire County Club to play there during the Australian winter in 2000. The reasons were more than financial. Even though Jane calls Australia home now, it would be good for her to spend some time with her family and friends, and being able to combine it with a season of county appealed to me. (The Australian Cricket Board had their reservations, saying they were scared I would burn myself out, but they could not actually stop me from going.) However, from the first day I knew I was going to become a father I insisted our baby would have to be born in Australia, and the reason for that is simple—I figured if we had a son there was no way on earth I'd let England claim him as a player! Jane didn't have a problem with this—she considers herself to be 100 per cent Australian now, and even her father, a proud Englishman, ignores the ribbing of his mates and supports the boys in green and gold too. The only person I have yet to convert is Jane's grandmother, and while she seems a tough nut to crack, I'm still trying.

WEDDING BELLS

J Ask any of the players' wives about organising their wedding and they'll tell you what a nightmare it is marrying a cricketer. You assume that once you've had the proposal you're home and dry, but trying to pin them down to a date is another story. Of course, it's not that they're not keen to see you walking down the aisle towards them, far from it. It's simply that the international cricket schedule is just so busy these days that it's really difficult to find a date in the calendar to fit the nuptials in. A couple of the girls have actually had to cancel their weddings when a tour has been arranged late in the day or their partner has been recalled to the side. It's all part and parcel of life as a 'cricket widow'.

Choosing my bridesmaids, in particular my Matron of Honour was one of the easiest tasks. Tracy Bevan is the sister I never had—ever since I first moved out to Australia, she's always been there for me. I also wanted my friend Lorraine. She'd started at Virgin at the same time as me, back in July 1989, and we'd been good friends ever since. Last, but by no means least, was Glenn's sister, Donna.

With Tracy's help, I had managed to get the most of the wedding organisation done before leaving for the West Indies—church, reception venue, invitations, flowers, etc, etc—leaving just the bare minimum to do in the three weeks we had after returning to Australia following the World Cup. My family were due to arrive the week before the wedding, as were Lorraine and her boyfriend Derek and also my friend Anna with her husband, Richard, and new baby girl, Emma, who were flying in from Hong Kong. I was thrilled that they were going to be at our wedding, but disappointed that I wasn't able to spend more time with them in the days before the wedding. It was just so hectic!

The week of our wedding the weather in Sydney was absolutely terrible. We had thunderstorms, lightning, torrential rain, gale force winds—I just couldn't believe it. Imagine my delight when on the Saturday morning, our big day, Tracy came into my bedroom with a cup of tea and told me to look out the window. She pulled the curtain back and the sunshine streamed in—it was the perfect start to a perfect day.

Our wedding day was one of the happiest days of my life and was filled with many unforgetable moments, but one of the most special came when I arrived at the church. The huge wooden doors were opened for the bridesmaids and my Dad and I to begin our walk down the aisle, and I saw that beautiful building filled with all of our family and friends and Glenn standing down at the altar waiting for me. It's a moment I shall always cherish. To be twelve weeks pregnant only made it more special. Most of our guests had to travel a fair distance to be at our wedding—from England, Hong Kong and interstate—and it meant so much to Glenn and me that they had made the effort to be there to share our wedding day. Their presence was the best wedding present of all.

WEDDING BELLS

G Few sporting teams have enjoyed the type of reception we received on our return to Australia. It seemed the public couldn't get enough of us—we were in demand at everything from functions to tickertape parades, and everywhere we went the world's greatest paperweight—the World Cup—accompanied us. In Melbourne and Sydney hundreds upon thousands of people lined the main streets to wave and cheer at us as we passed by in our cavalcade of open-topped cars. The view from the passenger's seat was extraordinary . . . a sea of happy and proud faces; banners with such messages as 'onya Aussies' and 'well done boys'; kids (some of them not so young) desperate to break through the security cordon and shake our hands and snare an autograph. The politicians were just as keen to meet the team with leaders from both sides of the political landscape jostling to be photographed with the players—especially our skipper. However, I had an even greater celebration on my mind: my wedding.

Jane had been left in charge of the details and she couldn't have done a better job. She kept the ceremony simple but it still had a fairytale touch, with the church she booked, the historic Garrison Church at The Rocks, and the reception centre, Curzon Hall, an old monastery. The Garrison's history stretches back to the early days of European settlement in Australia. It is made of local sandstone and furnished with shields from some of Australia's most famous military units from both World Wars. The church looks as if it could have been packed up and shipped over from Jane's homeland, and she was sold on it from the moment she saw the Union Jack and Australian flags hanging alongside each other behind the altar. She thought it was symbolic.

I asked Steve Waugh to be my Best Man because we've been through so much together; especially batting practice. (You see, Steve used to have the notion that not only was a batsman trapped in my body, he was screaming to get out. However, after many, many hard sessions he formed the conclusion that a stocking had more runs in it than my bat.) My brother Dale and cousin Craig made the big trip from the outback to be my groomsmen while in the blue corner, Jane had asked Tracy Bevan, my sister, Donna, and Lorraine Mutton to be her bridesmaids and, boy, they looked the part. While the wedding not only allowed my clan to meet Jane's family for the first time, it also gave us an opportunity to have all our friends under the one roof. When I went through the names on our invitation list, I couldn't help but feel there was plenty of quality there — decent, good people. There were friends from my childhood, members of the Sutherland, New South Wales and Australian sides, mates I have made since moving to the Big Smoke and Jane's circle of friends, some of whom she met during her battle with cancer.

Steve, Craig, Dale and I said farewell to my bachelorhood at Star City casino at Darling Harbour while Jane and the girls turned our house into a fortress. Jane is a brilliant organiser, and I certainly missed her magic touch the morning of the wedding. Before I embark on an overseas tour, or even a domestic match, Jane has this wonderful ability to find such things as my missing cricket trousers, boots and mobile telephone charger. Well, I can tell you we needed her help the morning of the big day because there was a litany of minor disasters, from shirts which didn't fit to groomsmen's shoes disappearing.

Merv Hughes, the former Test bowler, had a ritual in which he would wake on the morning of a game and look through a crack in the curtains to see what the weather was going to be like, and I did the same on my wedding day, 17 July.

Thankfully, the sky was a brilliant blue, there wasn't a cloud to be seen, and it was one of Sydney's trademark crisp winter days. However, it was nowhere near as perfect as Jane. When I saw her enter the church, I knew I had never been more right about anything in my life than marrying her. I had to catch my breath because she looked so beautiful; like a fairytale princess. The *Sunday Telegraph* said of Jane's arrival in a vintage Jaguar: WEARING A ROMANTIC, SLEEVELESS TULLE GOWN BEADED AT THE NECK WITH A HALF VEIL HELD BY A DELICATE TIARA, JANE ENTERED THE GARRISON CHURCH JUST A FEW MINUTES LATE TO MARRY THE MAN SHE CALLS 'HER ROCK'. She was actually about twenty minutes late but I didn't worry. I knew there was no way she would miss the ceremony . . . and when she finally lobbed the minister started and he was on fire. He really made the blokes in the congregation sit bolt upright during his sermon, which was about love and marriage, when he boomed: 'I know that in this church there is at least one man who does not love his wife!' That man, he said, must change. Thankfully, everyone didn't turn and look at this alleged man, whoever he may have been.

And then I looked into Jane's eyes and said 'I do'. They were the easiest two words to have ever passed my lips. We sealed our union with a kiss and began the long walk to the rest of our lives accompanied by the beautiful strains of the church organ and a shower of soap bubbles which the congregation blew from little plastic bottles. It was like walking on air.

Tracy Bevan was the star of the reception . . . her speech was hilarious, and she gave a unique insight into the secret which has made the Australian team such a dominant force. It had nothing to do with the slashing blade of her husband, Michael, the leadership of Steve Waugh, the wizard-like skills of Shane Warne or the efforts of our pace attack. No, with a dramatic movement she revealed Jane's 'lucky knickers', which she wears during a Test or a one-dayer. While Jane almost died of embarrassment, it was a definite highlight. Then my Best

Man, Steve Waugh, who met his wife, Lynette, when he was a shy 17-year-old at Sydney's East Hills Boys High, strode to the crease and offered some words of wisdom. Even on my greatest day he couldn't resist bringing up my well-known struggles with the bat: 'Jane and Glenn are a great couple, really well matched, with similar personalities, and very popular among their friends. I'm sure they'll have a great partnership together—better than his batting, I hope!' He added, 'They look really happy today. I've never seen them argue, which is pretty amazing, but obviously they will now that they're married. Any tips for marriage? It's like everything—keep working at it, Glenn, keep working at it.'

And I intend to. I don't really feel any different from before I was married, probably because we were so much in love. I know I have said it a few times already, but I do feel as though I have been charmed. That feeling was definitely with me two months after our wedding, on 17 September 1999—the second anniversary of Jane's operation. When I look at the way our life has turned around since that dark time I can't help but feel we'll beat any future challenges which might present themselves in the future. We're a team.

A DREAM COME TRUE

J The day I gave birth to our son James, 20 January 2000, was the best day of my life. He looked so perfect and beautiful—he was a little miracle, the most precious thing in the world.

One of the worst things about being told I had breast cancer was also being warned that I might never be able to have children. Having a family was something that I'd always just taken for granted—of course I'd have kids one day. The prospect of not being about to fulfil this dream left me feeling completely and utterly devastated. But I just took one step at a time, determined to give my body every possible chance to beat both the cancer and the threat of infertility. I drank my juices religiously, took all the recommended vitamins and anti-oxidants and, most importantly, remained positive. That the chemotherapy didn't cause my periods to stop I took as a very good sign. My oncologist had recommended that we wait at least twelve months after the last chemo session (in April 1998) before trying for a baby to give my body a chance to recover from the onslaught of drugs that had been running through my veins.

Glenn and I both wanted to have children sooner rather than later, so when the twelve months were up, we decided that we'd start trying. It wasn't really a conscious effort to get pregnant, more of a 'well, let's go about our business and see what happens!' sort of thing. We thought it could take months, maybe years for me to fall, so we had nothing to lose by giving it a go. The way things worked out, I fell pregnant almost as soon as I arrived in Barbados!

I had a fantastic pregnancy. Hardly any morning sickness in those first three months—certainly nothing that I could complain about. I felt fit and well from May up until Christmas, which was when the fluid settled in everywhere and I felt like a beached whale. It just seemed to creep up on me—one day I felt great and the next morning, I looked in the mirror and saw a face like a full moon staring back at me. A good night's sleep quickly became a thing of the past—and it probably will be for the next twenty years. James was a very active baby inside me; he never seemed to stop kicking and moving around. Now I've seen he's got his Dad's long legs I know why.

James was originally due on 4 February—the date of the second One Day Final in Sydney. However, as my pregnancy progressed, I was convinced that he'd be coming early. Everyone kept on telling me not to worry, that your first baby generally arrives late, but I was sure that this one wouldn't. My obstetrician, Margaret, came highly recommended to me by Lynette Waugh and was a keen follower of cricket. She was also accustomed to the problems of fitting a birth into a hectic cricket schedule. After much discussion with Margaret regarding James' due date and Glenn's schedule, we decided that in order to guarantee Glenn being present at the birth (which was something that he and I both very much wanted), she would induce me on 20 January, the day immediately following a one-day match at the SCG. The baby would be 38 weeks along.

A few days before this, I started having cramps and feeling generally very uncomfortable. Even just walking around, I felt as though I could give birth at any moment. Glenn and I were told to be at the hospital at 7 o'clock on the morning of 20 January. The midwife had a look at me and informed me that I was already 2 cm dilated. She said that rather than put any gel on my cervix, my obstetrician would probably choose to break my waters and get things underway, which is precisely what happened when she arrived at 7.45 am. I was told to get some rest in preparation for the pushing I would have to do later that afternoon. I was too excited to sleep but Glenn lay down on a sofa in the corner of the delivery suite and managed to get a couple of hours rest in. After forty-five minutes of pushing, which I would liken to pushing a truck uphill and then being told you have to push it round the corner, little James entered the world at 3.24 pm, weighing 3 kg (7 lbs 2 ½ oz) and measuring 51 cm. I felt totally overwhelmed with love for him and bursting with pride—it was the most amazing experience of my life. I'd do it again tomorrow!

I'd been hoping I'd still be able to breastfeed, and now the moment of truth had arrived. Of course I only had the one side from which to feed my baby, and I prayed my milk would come through and that James would take it. I can't describe my feelings when I first fed him—he took to the breast straight away. And my milk supply has been amazing. It's incredible to me how my body has healed itself: not only has it recovered from a life-threatening disease, but it's gone on to create and sustain another life, another human being. That just blows me away.

I look at James and my heart melts. One smile from him

makes everything in my life right. I'd been told I might never have children and now we've been blessed with our own little miracle. My life is a dream come true.

G A bloke can think he's seen a lot of life—I've gazed at some of the great natural wonders of the world—but nothing, and I mean nothing, is anywhere near as humbling as laying eyes on your newborn child. When little James Sidney McGrath entered the world at 3.24 pm on 20 January I felt a mixture of emotions. I felt love, a desire to protect him and a desire to meet each and every need of this little fellow and my wife; it was an incredible emotional surge and I'd never felt anything like it before. While Jane did all the hard work—and it was tough, because she'd opted for a natural birth—I cut the umbilical chord, and felt an instant, incredible bond with my son. It was the greatest feeling imaginable, and gave me an intense feeling of warmth and love. I've heard some fathers say they have almost fainted while witnessing the birth of their child, but I was too mesmerised to feel anything but a genuine fascination. I saw his head coming— he had a dark crop of hair—and when I looked up at Jane panting, sweating and straining I thought, 'this is it, we're going to become parents'. And then, with an almighty final push, he was born. I cut the cord and the doctor placed James straight on Jane's chest where he wailed his little lungs out . . . perhaps we have an opera singer on our hands. I noticed a lot of Jane in his features straight away, though I could see he'd inherited his Dad's long and skinny legs. It's my great hope that those legs carry him on some great adventures through his life.

Actually, I think James will be one of those kids who throw themselves head first into life—he was in one heck of a rush to see the world and he hasn't slowed down since.

A DREAM COME TRUE

I hope I've made it crystal clear throughout this book that I have nothing but admiration for Jane's fighting qualities . . . and James' birth is a testimony to her courage and determination. When the doctors said Jane might not be able to have children because of the drugs that were needed to fight the breast cancer she didn't give up hope of becoming a mother. When we decided to try and have a family we were told there was nothing to worry about from the chemicals which had been used to beat the cancer, but the doctors went to great pains to explain there was a strong chance their after-affects could have left her barren . . . but she didn't wave the white flag. I didn't have immediate plans to start a family, that was Jane's idea, but now that we have the little fellow I appreciate how much poorer we were without him.

One thing which amazed me about James' birth was that while we didn't speak to the media I've been told news of his arrival was on the radio within the hour. It's frightening, and what was even worse were the lucrative offers we received to 'sell' the story of his birth to local and overseas publications. Although we had agreed to sell the story of our wedding to a magazine—in the hope it would mean that the event was less likely to be crashed by other media—there was no way we'd do it in this case. It was too precious a time and we wanted some privacy.

My cricket commitments kept me away from Jane and James during his first few months because no sooner had we wrapped up the World Series Cup against Pakistan than we were dispatched to New Zealand for a two-month tour, followed by a lightning trip to South Africa to compete in a one-day tournament. But they were always on my mind, and in the time we were together I felt so protective of the little guy that I'd carry him, I'd push the pram, I'd cuddle him, I'd change his nappy. I was so proud to be his father, and the sad experience of being separated from him and his mother gave me an awful insight into the sense of lost time Mark Taylor, Steve Waugh and Ian Healy complained of during their trips away to cricket's far-flung outposts. It's funny how James has also changed Jane's outlook on motherhood—now she is talking about having three kids!

A few days after James' birth I was named the inaugural recipient of the Allan Border Medal in recognition for my efforts with the Australian side during the previous twelve months. It was a great thrill for a number of reasons. Being the first to win the Border medal is incredible because no matter who wins it next year, or even in a century's time, I'll always have been the first. It was also a great thrill because Allan was my first Test skipper. I'll always remember my first encounter with the grumpy old bull doing his best to put a young turk off his game. We locked horns in a Sheffield Shield match and I frustrated his attempts to sledge me by ignoring him and remaining silent. (He ultimately gave up.) Less than a decade later I had a medal with his name around my neck and was searching for the words to describe my emotions. Hearing Richie Benaud describe me as one of the finest bowlers ever to represent Australia was humbling, but my thoughts were with Jane and James back at home in our lounge room with Lynette Waugh keeping them company. I told the crowd of my love and admiration for Jane, and while there was a lot of feeling in my voice I don't think I did justice to the depth of my passion for her . . . words just don't do it.

A DREAM COME TRUE

I'm a lucky man. I'm not overly religious, but I know God has blessed me, truly blessed me, for reasons only He knows. When Jane was diagnosed with breast cancer it tore at my heart because I saw the terrible fear in her eyes. Apart from offering my wholehearted support and unconditional love there was nothing more I could do. We saw it through together and I'm a better person for it. When Jane made it clear she would prefer to die than lose her breast I couldn't understand how she could give up . . . it was only later that I came to realise that Jane needed to sink to the depths of her despair before she could appreciate the beauty of life. I get a lot of strength on a daily basis from Jane and I hope people who read this book gain some of it through reading about her will—and her frailties. Ignorance and fear is the real killer. Breast cancer is an evil, twisted, son-of-a-bitch but it doesn't necessarily mean the end of life as you know it. Life can actually get better; I know it has for Jane and me. We have a full life in every sense, and now that we have little James I know it is only going to get even better and richer.

If your partner is suffering from breast cancer you have my support and prayers. Be brave. Be supportive and, if you're strong enough, don't run. Your woman needs you now more than ever.

Just remember, as I learned, true love can help conquer all.

EPILOGUE

J When Random House approached us with the idea of writing a book together about our experience of breast cancer I was adamant that if we agreed to do it then it had to be a brutally honest, true-to-life account, otherwise it was pointless. I haven't sugar-coated anything because that would give a false impression. Battling breast cancer isn't easy; it's one of the toughest challenges you could ever face, and you need all the inner strength, courage and support that you can possibly muster.

For those of you reading this whose lives have been affected by breast cancer, and especially those of you who are fighting it now, we wrote this book for you. I know first-hand how incredibly frightening it can be to be diagnosed with breast cancer, but I want you to know that it doesn't automatically mean a death sentence. If I can beat it, so can you.

All women should be breast aware: look out for any puckering, changes in shape or size, inverted or flaking nipples. Know every millimetre of your breasts—90 per cent of breast cancers are discovered by women themselves, as mine

EPILOGUE

was. Trust your instincts. If you suspect that something just isn't quite right, take a deep breath and do something about it: nine out of ten lumps are not cancerous. Go and see your GP—a problem shared is a problem halved.

It angers me that mammograms are mainly targeted at women over fifty. I realise that breast tissue in younger women is denser and so mammograms are harder to interpret but that doesn't mean it's impossible to spot a problem and so as far as I'm concerned, younger women should be encouraged to have them, especially as tumours tend to spread faster in young women. Surely it's better to be safe than sorry. I was told by one specialist that my lumps may have been growing undetected for three or four years. Statistics stating that women under fifty are at an extremely low risk of getting the disease are of little consolation to those of us under fifty who have been diagnosed with it. Early detection is vital, so don't waste a second. Your health is in your hands.

Five years ago I never would have believed in my wildest dreams that I'd end up living in Australia, married to my gorgeous best friend, living in a fabulous waterfront home with our beautiful son. I also would never have believed that I'd lose a breast to cancer and live to tell the tale. I guess that's what makes life so amazing—you just never know what's around the corner. One of the many things I've learned from my recent experience is that you should live life to the fullest, make the most of every single day and remember that each day that dawns is a great day to be alive.

ACKNOWLEDGEMENTS

Of all the people we'd like to thank in connection with our book the first has to be Hazel Flynn at Random House, who approached us with the idea with so much enthusiasm it was impossible to say no to her. There wouldn't be a book if it weren't for her. Thank you Hazel, and also Katie Stackhouse at Random House for your support and advice. Huge thanks also to Daniel Lane who, when not out dolphin spotting, managed to find time to assist Glenn with his half of our story.

If it weren't for Dr Anthony Ethell, Professor John Kearsley, Dr Kiran Phadke and Dr Chris Hughes I may not have been around to write my side of the story and I will forever be indebted to them for their medical expertise and support.

Thank you Mrs Bevan, not only for being my best friend but also for being a great sounding board. To Mum, Dad and Jon, I'm so grateful for your encouragement and confidence in my ability to do a good job! Extra-special thanks to Mum for being such a fantastic role model, for taking such great care of baby James enabling me to get stuck into the final stages of writing, for somehow keeping me calm when the disk containing hours of work became corrupt overnight and finally for the endless cups of Earl Grey which kept the ink and inspiration flowing!

WHAT SHOULD I LOOK OUT FOR?

This is the latest advice from the National Breast Cancer Centre.

Look for any changes in your breasts which are not normal for you, or which you haven't seen before. You should see your GP about the following important changes:

- **a lump, lumpiness or thickening.** For younger women—if this is not related to your normal monthly cycle and remains after your period. For women of all ages—if this is a new change in one breast only.

- **changes to the nipple.** Such as a change in shape, crusting, a sore or an ulcer, redness or indrawing of the nipple.

- **discharge from the nipple.** If this is from one nipple and is bloodstained, or occurs without squeezing.

- **changes in the skin of a breast.** Such as any puckering or dimpling of the skin, unusual redness or other colour change.

- **persistent, unusual pain.** If this is not related to your normal monthly cycle, remains after your period and occurs in one breast only.

- **a change in the shape or size of a breast.** This might be either an increase or a decrease in size.

Knowing what is normal for you is just as important after menopause because breast cancer becomes more common as you grow older.

CONTACTS & RESOURCES

National Cancer Organisations
Cancer Information Service (CIS)
A telephone counselling and information service on all cancer and cancer related issues.
Toll-free number: 1800 422 760
For callers outside Sydney: 131 120 (except QLD)
For Sydney metropolitan area: (02) 9334 1933
TTY (for the hearing impaired): (02) 9334 1865
For those who require assistance with information in their own language, the CIS will link to the Translating and Interpreting Service (TIS).

National Breast Cancer Centre (NBBC)
Managed by the NSW Cancer Council, the NBBC's aim is to disseminate accurate and accessible information about breast cancer. It also has a special responsibility to improve access to information and services for women and health professionals living in rural and remote areas of Australia and from non-English speaking, Aboriginal and Torres Strait Island backgrounds. The comprehensive website has a wealth of information available, including a detailed list of resources and further reading, plus links to other useful websites, both Australian and overseas.
NSW Cancer Council
4th floor, 153 Dowling Street
Woolloomooloo, NSW 2011
Mail: PO Box 572, Kings Cross NSW 1340
Ph: (02) 9334 1700; Fax: (02) 9326 9329
E-mail: directorate@nbcc.org.au
Website: www.nbcc.org.au

Breastscreen Australia
Breastscreen Australia aims to help women over the age of 50 to detect breast cancer at an early stage, and to find cancers that are too small to feel. For more information about mammographic screening services in your area, phone 132 050 for the cost of a local call.

CONTACTS AND RESOURCES

Breast Cancer Network Australia (BCNA)
The BCNA is the national voice of Australians personally affected by breast cancer. The BCNA publishes The Beacon, *a national newsletter for women with breast cancer.*
The national coordinator
PO Box 4082
Auburn South VIC 3122
Ph: (03) 9805 2500; Fax: (03) 9805 2599
Email: beacon@bcna.org.au
Website: www.bcna.org.au

State and Territory Cancer Organisations
Contact the following head offices for information about regional offices.

ACT Cancer Society Inc.
159 Maribyrnong Avenue
Kaleen ACT 2617
Ph: (02) 6262 2222; Fax: (02) 6262 2223
Email: actcancer@cancer.org.au

NSW Cancer Council
153 Dowling Street
Woolloomooloo NSW 2011
Mail: PO Box 572
Kings Cross NSW 1340
Ph: (02) 9334 1900; Fax: (02) 9357 2676
TTY: (02) 9334 1865
or 1800 422 760 (outside Sydney)
Website: www.nswcc.org.au

Cancer Council of the Northern Territory
Casi House, 3/23 Vanderlin Drive
Casuarina NT 0810
Mail: PO Box 42719
Casuarina NT 0811
Ph: (08) 8927 4888 or 1800 678 123 (outside Darwin)
Fax: (08) 8927 4990
Website: www.cancercouncil.citysearch.au

Queensland Cancer Fund
553 Gregory Terrace
Fortitude Valley QLD 4006
Ph: (07) 3258 2200; Fax: (07) 3257 1306
Email: qldcf@qldcancer.com.au
Website: www.qldcancer.com.au

Anti-Cancer Foundation of South Australia
202 Greenhill Road
Eastwood SA 5063
Mail: PO Box 929
Unley SA 5061
Ph: (08) 8291 4111 or 1800 188 070 (outside Adelaide)
Fax: (08) 8291 4122
Website: www.cancersa.org.au

Cancer Council of Tasmania
140 Bathurst Street
Hobart TAS 7000
Ph: (03) 6233 2030; Fax: (03) 6233 2123
Website: www.tased.edu.au/tasonline/cancer/cancer.htm

PO Box 1864
Shop 2 Jimmy's Shopping Complex
216 Charles Street
Launceston TAS 7250
Ph: (03) 6336 2030; Fax: (03) 6336 2789
Website: www.tased.edu.au/tasonline/cancer/cancer.htm

Anti-Cancer Council of Victoria
1 Rathdowne Street
Carlton South VIC 3053
Cancer Helpline: 131 120 (from anywhere in Victoria)
Ph: (03) 9635 5000; Fax: (03) 9635 5270
Email: enquiries@accv.org.au
Website: www.accv.org.au

CONTACTS AND RESOURCES

Cancer Foundation of Western Australia
334 Rokeby Road
Subiaco WA 6008
Ph: (08) 9381 4515; Fax: (08) 9381 4523
Website: www.cancerwa.asn.au

Breast Cancer Support Groups
National Cancer Information Line
Phone 131 120 from anywhere in Australia for the cost of a local phone call for information about cancer and to find out about support services in your state or territory, or visit the NBCC website: www.nbcc.org.au

Breast Cancer Support Service (BCSS)
The BCSS is a national service coordinated by the state and territory cancer organisations which aims to provide practical and emotional support to women diagnosed with breast cancer. Volunteers can speak with women over the phone or can arrange a visit. The service is confidential and free. Phone the national cancer information line 131 120 (1300 360 366 in Queensland) or the BCSS coordinator at your state or territory cancer organisation.

Look Good ... Feel Better
A community service for women undergoing cancer treatment, dedicated to teaching women beauty techniques to help restore their appearance and self-image during chemotherapy and radiotherapy. For information about workshops, contact:
'Look Good ... Feel Better' National Helpline: 1800 650 960

The Lymphoedema Association of Australia Inc.
Has information and links to state and territory support groups.
94 Cambridge Terrace
Malvern SA 5061
Ph: (08) 8271 2198; Fax: (08) 8271 8776
Email: casley@enternet.com.au
Website: www.lymphoedema.org.au

Jane's Recommendations
Mastectomy bras and swimwear
Amoena
Amoena products are available in Australia through various retailers. For your nearest retailer:
Ph: 1800 773 285 (freecall)
Website: www.coloplast.com.au

Nicola Jane
Ph: (0011 44) 1243 790900 (for catalogue and to order)
Website: www.nicolajane.co.uk

Reading
Clinkard, C. E., *The Uses of Juices: Extracted from raw fruits and vegetables*, Penguin New Zealand, 1980.

Note: This information was correct at the time of writing.